WILDFIRE WITHIN

RISING FROM THE ASHES

CHANTAL RUSSELL

Published by The Well Publishing, November 2017
ISBN: 9781775034902

Copyright © 2017 by Chantal Russell
All rights reserved. No part of this publication may be reproduced, stored in, or introduced into a retrieval system, or transmitted, in any form, or by any means (electronic, mechanical, photocopying, recording, or otherwise) without the prior written permission of the publisher. This book is sold subject to the condition that it shall not, by way of trade or otherwise, be lent, resold, hired out, or otherwise circulated without the publisher's prior consent in any form of binding or cover other than that in which it is published, and without a similar condition including this condition being imposed on the subsequent purchaser.

Editor: Nina Shoroplova
Typeset: Greg Salisbury
Book Cover Design: Naomi MacDougall
Portrait Photographer: Britney Gill Photography

DISCLAIMER: Some names and identifying details have been changed to protect the privacy of individuals. This book is not intended as a substitute for the medical advice of physicians. The reader should regularly consult a physician in matters relating to his/her health and particularly with respect to any symptoms that may require diagnosis or medical attention.

To my Mother, my Grand-Mothers,
and the Great Mother who nourishes us all

Acknowledgements

So many have contributed to the creation of this book. I want to thank Gary, my amazing husband and soul partner, who continues to love and support me, no matter where my wild dreams seem to take us. Thank you for being the steady riverbank to my Shakti soul river.

Thank you to my mother Francine and sister Nicole; you are my Guadalupe Angels and I could never have gotten through the dark nights without your unwavering love and support. Thank you to my father Gerry and my brother Steph for being there and always accepting me exactly as I am.

Thank you to Sianna Sherman, my teacher, my mentor, my deep soul friend. The many hours we have spent together have enriched my life, and I owe much of the wisdom gleaned from my experiences to you. I have so much love and ever-flowing gratitude for your presence in my life.

I want to thank my amazing soul sisters who continue to inspire me. Laura Larriva Page a.k.a. Shakti Sunfire: Thank you from the bottom of my heart for bringing moon magic into my life at such a pivotal time. Your guidance helped me become whole again. To Marni Sclaroff and Kaitlyn Baptist: Thank you for the countless soul sessions. All the tears and laughs we've shared have been holy and so healing.

To Rosemary, Nancy, and Esteban, my Costa Rican soul family, thank you for welcoming me into your homes and opening my eyes and heart to the spirit and beauty of *pura vida*.

Thank you to Nicholas Callaway, Amanda Giacomini, and MC Yogi for your loving words of encouragement and for always reminding me that I have something worthwhile to share. Without your loving nudges, I would not have had the courage to write this book.

Thank you to Julie Salisbury, Nina Shoroplova, and Naomi

MacDougall for holding my hand and helping me birth this book baby into the world. I'm grateful to each of you for your skillful artistry.

To you my dear reader, thank you for the gift of your time and attention. May my story serve to liberate and empower you to enjoy your precious life, and become the heroine of your own sacred journey.

And to Ben, my beloved boy. This book would not have been possible without you. I love you to Chiron and back.

Contents

Dedication iii
Acknowledgements v
Prologue xi

Chapter 1: Spark: Giving Birth 1
    Full Moon 1
    Life Spark 2
    Birth 4
    Death 8
    The Call 11
    Meditation and Medication 12
    Contraction and Expansion 20
    Pulse and Flow 25

Chapter 2: Flames: You Will Find a Way 27
    The Disseminating Moon 27
    The Space Between 28
    View from the Top 30
    Wandering into Yoga 33
    Mother India 34
    You Will Find a Way 42
    Converse with God 45
    The Flow of Grace 46
    The Earth Is Quaking 51

Chapter 3: Embers: Learning to Let Go 57
    Last Quarter Moon 57
    Chicago in the Autumn 58
    Rooting Down 61
    Becoming a Householder 64
    Follow the Dream 67

    The Householder's Path 68
    Remembering My Own Light 71
    From Tadasana to Savasana 73
    The Tomb Is the Womb 76
    Surrender 77

Chapter 4: Ashes: Dying to be Free 81
    The Balsamic Moon 81
    The Heart of Recognition 84
    This Is Happening for You 89
    La Vie En Soul 91
    Becoming Soul Fluent 92

Chapter 5: Rebirth: Embrace the Dark 98
    New Moon 98
    Snake Medicine 99
    Dark Days of the Soul 99
    The Girl with the Feather Tattoo 102
    Surrender Some More 105
    Mantra Medicine 106
    Twice Born 110
    Salt Water Cures 112
    Awakening Desire 116
    Sweat It Out 119
    Savour the Flavours 120
    Releasing the Good Girl 121
    Receive the Gift 123
    Holy, Healthy, Whole 124

Chapter 6: Cherish the Seed: Explore Your Potential 126
    Crescent Moon 126
    Aligning with the Moon 131
    Stay Wild 133

The Circle 134
Nature's Design 135
Be Your Own Heroine.. 138
The Five Layers: Your Five Bodies 141
Your Body is the Living Vessel 145
Don't Mistake the Map for the Journey................................... 149

Chapter 7: Nourish the Root: Nurture Your Nature 151
First Quarter Moon.. 151
Becoming a Conscious Creator 152
Be a Creator, Not a Reactor.. 153
Soul and Spirit.. 155
Nourish Your Soul.. 156
Become Soul-Centric... 157

Chapter 8: Tend to the Shoot: Embody Freedom 160
Gibbous Moon 160
Vibrant Health.. 161
Grow Roots and Wings.. 163
Stoke the Digestive Fire 166
Tend to the Heart Fire... 167
The Beauty Way 168
Cultivate Radiance 170
Weave Thyself 172
Cross the Threshold 174
Your Life Is Your Craft 176
More Soul Alignment, Less Daily Grind................................... 177

Chapter 9: Flourish: Bloom Wildly 179
The Full Moon Always Returns... 179
The Dark Feminine 180
Remember to Remember... 183
Perfectly Imperfect 185

Created to Create 187
Your Desires Become Your Destiny 188
Wildfire 191
Redwoods 192
Wild Flowers 193
Be Your Own Midwife 194
Savasana 195

Author Biography 197
Contact The Author 198
Appendix 1 199
Appendix 2 200
Appendix 3 201

Prologue

"As if you were on fire from within, the moon lives in the lining of your skin." Pablo Neruda

Each of us is on our own unique heroine's journey, a quest to discover what we're made of, and to understand why we're here.

In 1955, while moving what appeared to be a very large stucco statue of the Buddha, Thai workers were amazed at what they miraculously discovered inside the ancient form. In the midst of holding the five-ton statue off its pedestal to transport it to a new palace home in Bangkok, the ropes broke from the sheer weight, causing the statue to fall to the ground. Upon landing, a piece of the sturdy stucco cracked off, exposing a luminous Golden Buddha underneath its outer casing.

Hundreds of years prior, the Siamese people had covered up their statue made of gold with plaster and stained glass, in an effort to hide its worth and keep it from being stolen by rivaling Burmese invaders. The statue remained hidden, and eventually its priceless value was forgotten for over two hundred years. Shortly after dropping the statue and breaking its shell, the Thai removed the remaining stucco to reveal the largest Golden Buddha in the entire world.

Like the radiant Golden Buddha, our core—our true nature—is luminous; but we have forgotten what lies within us. The heroine's journey we are each on is not an outward quest for a Holy Grail, but an inward journey to the core of who we are. That core, our soul, is the innermost layer of ourself, and the one we are here to reveal in this lifetime. What we're truly made of has been buried beneath the surface, suppressed from our awareness, and ignored for far too long.

The heroine's journey is essentially a journey to the centre of our being, to our innermost Golden Buddha nature. It is the pilgrimage we must all take to discover what we're made of. The hardships we experience serve not to break us down, but to break us open. The wildfires come not to destroy us, but to consume anything that is keeping us from remembering who we really are. Just as the bird must break through its shell to live into its full potential, we must trust the wildfire flames that come to devour all that we are not.

Joy and the wellbeing we seek come not from controlling the external circumstances of our life but from aligning with who we really are. True health can only emerge when we attune to the purpose of our existence; when we embody the one we came here to be; and when we share the soul gift we alone carry for others.

The moon has long been a symbol of the soul. To unearth the golden soul radiance within, we can look to nature and the cycles of the moon to understand ourselves more deeply. During my own path to healing from cancer, learning about the moon phases became an empowering reflection of my own soul's evolutionary journey. Seeing how she emerges from darkness to light, then back to darkness every month, I came to understand more deeply the nourishment of night, the necessity of death, the power of rebirth, and my own cyclic nature. To experience the vibrant health and vitality I so deeply longed for, I needed to re-member that, like the moon, I am wild and whole, and ever changing.

Re-wilding myself back to wholeness has been about rediscovering the magic of nature. By magic, I mean a shift of perspective so that I could see the *extra* ordinary in the ordinary, witness the innate patterns found throughout all of creation, and discover the miraculous Universe at play through my own life. The moon was my portal back to the ways of nature.

Every twenty-eight days the moon moves through eight phases that are symbolic of seasons, our own life cycle, and the heroine's soul journey we each find ourselves on.

Whether we are healing our body, our relationships, or are simply looking to awaken our wild creativity, the moon's wisdom offers us guidance along our own heroine's journey:

The Full Moon: Shine, play, dance, rise, be passionate, love, celebrate, forgive
Disseminating Moon: Gather, relax, accept, understand, regroup, wander
Last Quarter Moon: Listen within, turn inward, reevaluate, reorient toward letting go
Balsamic Moon: Let go, trust fate, meditate, heal, soothe, rest, breathe
The New Moon: Plant, intuit, open, tell the truth, dream, surrender, release
The Crescent Moon: Step out, mobilize, hope, have faith, reach, begin
First Quarter Moon: Activate, build, risk, be confident, plunge in, promise, commit
Gibbous Moon: Clarify, persevere, ask, design, tweak, hone, adjust, expand

Learning about each of these phases helped me re-align my body and soul to its innate wholeness. Understanding nature's rhythm gave me permission to slow down, recalibrate at the deepest level, and dream anew. For me, true healing began when I learned to embrace the dark side of the moon; when I came to trust the Dark Feminine; and when I truly understood the transformative power of the eternal flame of love.

CHAPTER ONE

Spark: Giving Birth (Full Moon)

Full Moon: Shine, play, dance, rise, be passionate, love, celebrate, forgive

"If you bring forth what is within you, what you bring forth will save you. If you do not bring forth what is within you, what you do not bring forth will destroy you." *Gospel of Thomas*

"Birth is the death of the life we have known; death, the birth of the life we have yet to live." Marion Woodman

"You never know how badly you want to live until you are faced with your death." Elisa Romeo

"Paradox is usually a sign of the presence of soul." Thomas Moore

Full Moon

During her brightest phase, the Full Moon symbolizes abundance, birth, and the energy of fire. Amidst the point of highest light in her most radiant expression, paradoxically, she begins her return to darkness. Like the full moon, the moment a labouring woman gives birth, simultaneously, is the moment when she needs to let go of the woman she has been, of the baby she has carried, and of the life she has known. The Full Moon reminds us that the fulfillment (fullness) we seek comes when we learn to let go.

There are many such full-moon moments throughout one's life, times when something new is created, and something old is released. Yet only few such flashes of light have the power to transform you forever. There are those wildfire full moon moments that mark your life for evermore; moments when you realize nothing will ever be the same and time is divided into two parts—before this and after this.

There is the visible life you live on the outside, of work and family and responsibilities; and the hidden life of dreams and desires and soul, which you keep unlived on the inside. It is in those full-moon threshold moments—of before this and after this—that the journey of finding and becoming oneself takes place.

If you choose to bring forth what is within you, what is within you will not only save you, but could light up the whole sky, and be the very spark needed to ignite a much-needed wildfire.

Although, outwardly, wildfires seem to leave only devastation in their wake, inwardly, wildfires—those crisis points where life seems to be falling apart, the before-this-and-after-this moments—are necessary and deeply beneficial for the growth and health of the forests which they devour.

Life Spark

In December 2011, I gave birth to my son Benjamin. A true celebration of love, it was the most beautiful, exhilarating,

Chapter One

and empowering experience of my life. But like a wildfire that ravaged the beauty around me, it was also one of the most devastating days of my life, one that I will never forget, and not for the reasons you may think.

Years before I was pregnant, I had taken prenatal yoga teacher training and discovered nature's optimal design for childbirth. After learning how medical interventions can throw the whole thing off course and only lead to needing more interventions down the line, I knew that when it was my time to become a mother, I would opt for a natural, unmedicated birth. I wanted to be totally awake and conscious, to witness the wild beauty of life, and to feel the power of being a woman. I intended to welcome my baby into the world and into my arms with clarity and full presence, and longed to feel the full spectrum of sensations and emotions that childbirth awakens. So when that time did come years later, when I became pregnant two years into my marriage, my husband Greg and I prepared for a home birth, and planned for the best.

Knowing that a conscious birth requires a loving support team, I asked my sister Nicole to be my doula. She flew to Vancouver in British Columbia (BC) from Toronto, Ontario near the time of my due date to assist at the birth. With my sister-doula, husband-support coach, and amazing midwives by my side, I felt ready and eager to become a mother. My due date of December 15 came and went and, knowing that I did not want to be induced on Christmas Day (if baby hasn't arrived ten days past your due date, they'll induce you), I was anxious to get things moving along. After a day of foot rubs, spicy foods, and ecstatic dancing, my water finally broke the next day on Friday December 16 around 11 p.m.; labour had officially begun! After the initial excitement and a little happy dance, both my sister and hubby went to bed, and slept through the night. I was too excited to sleep, so I stayed up clearing my inbox as I bounced on an exercise ball between contractions.

At the time, I was apprenticing with and managing world-renowned yoga teacher, Sianna Sherman, booking her flights and photo shoots, connecting and coordinating events with people all over the world, and assisting her at festivals and conferences globally.

Three months before my due date, I had been in Paris with the team assisting at a yoga teacher training. One of my best friends, Rheana lived in Paris at the time, working for Christian Louboutin, the famous shoe designer. While in Paris, my love of French fashion trumped my comfort-loving inner-hippie mama. I happily forced my swollen pregnant feet into red-soled six-inch heels, and walked to teacher training in Louby's every day.

The week after that, we were in New York doing a photoshoot, working with Madonna's publisher, who snapped a shot of me doing a handstand on the rooftop of a high rise in Union Square, at six months pregnant. The yoga world I found myself in was full of hustle, glamour, and Grace. It was busy, things moved fast, and I loved it.

Birth

In between contractions, after answering all lingering emails, I put an autoresponder that read, "Away having a baby, will respond in two weeks, thanks for your patience," I shut down my computer, and sat on the couch.

The contractions were intensifying. I started moaning. Loudly. My sister woke up around 6 a.m. because she could hear my groans. With not much else to do but be, relax, and let things happen on their own, we watched *Dirty Dancing*, one of our favourite movies since growing up in the 1980s. We laughed

Chapter One

at how inappropriate it was for our parents to let us watch it back in the day as young children, but also thought it was mildly empowering that they did. "Nobody puts Baby in the corner" should be every girl's mantra.

The midwives came over later that morning, and left shortly after to attend at another birth, when they assessed that I was only four centimetres dilated.

"We'll come back this afternoon and stay when she's six centimetres dilated, in more active labour," they told my sister-husband birth team. Since I was still in early labour at only four centimetres, they knew we still had a few hours before things really started moving.

"How will we know she's in 'active labour'?" Greg asked.

The lovely midwives explained that in the early stages of labour, a woman is coherent and able to maintain a conversation in between contractions. When she enters the later stage of labour, she is immersed in another world—this is "active labour." When the intensity of sensation plus the cocktail of hormones take over her body and logic is no longer present, a woman enters the primal galaxy from where she came. She goes into a trancelike state where the logical part of the brain (the neocortex) is no longer in charge. She moves into her deep, primal, ancient brain (the limbic system) where the body knows what to do without conscious thinking and planning. She is taken over by Shakti, the creative power of the Universe, Mother Nature herself.

"You'll know it when you see it," they assured him, smiling as they left our tiny twenty-third floor, Yaletown apartment.

The contractions continued to intensify. When the midwives came back a few hours later, I was seven centimetres dilated. I took a bath to relax, and Greg held my hand to support me through the contractions.

While soaking in the tub, I remembered Gisele Bündchen,

my female supermodel crush, in a birth documentary I had seen her in weeks earlier. She had described her birth contractions as being like waves cresting and falling. I invoked my inner Gisele and pictured the contractions as though they were warm Costa Rican ocean waves, rolling in, cresting over me, then rolling out. Each painful peak was followed by a moment of bliss.

In all of the books I had read during pregnancy (*Ina May's Guide to Natural Childbirth*, *HypnoBirthing*, and my favourite, *Orgasmic Birth*), the authors explained that although birth is "intense," the female body is equipped to meet the increasing discomfort of labour by progressively releasing feel-good hormones, such as oxytocin and endorphins. In fact, in hypnobirthing circles, they don't even use the word "pain," because it has a negative connotation in our culture. According to these wonderful mamas, there is no word in the English language to accurately and positively describe the sensation of childbirth. Instead, they use words like "pressure" and "surges" to convey the movements of energy.

In an unmedicated birth, each contraction—each surge—is followed by a burst of oxytocin, and feelings of bliss and euphoria, in a pulsatile, gradually increasing, perfectly timed way. In other words, as labour progresses and your contractions become more intense, your body creates and releases increasing amounts of the feel-good hormones to meet and mediate the increasing intensity of the experience. The key is to let the discomfort happen and not numb the pain. If you choose to take something to dull the pain, it will also dull the pleasure. Let it happen, feel the energy move through you, and you will be suffused with natural opiates and showered with sensations of elation. Innate powers you didn't know you had will be activated.

While I was pregnant, I was very discerning about the books I read and the media I ingested. In prenatal yoga training, I

Chapter One

was introduced to the growing field of perinatal and prenatal psychology, which proves how our early experiences inside the womb affect not only our development as a fetus, but will set into motion patterns that will play out in the rest of our lives. While in the womb, babies are marinating in the flavours of their mother's experience. Whatever mama feels, baby feels. If mama is stressed or fearful after arguing with someone for example, baby will respond by being in a heightened state of stress *in utero*, and will be more prone to experience fear and stress as a natural state once outside the womb, more biologically wired to pick a fight. From early on, we are being shaped by our environment and shown that we live in a malleable Universe, one that responds to the choices we make.

During my labour, in the midst of a particularly strong contraction, I leaned my head back and clenched my teeth with a strong breath in through the narrow opening of my lips, to bear the intensity. Greg noticed a strange lump just above my collarbone, framed by the awkward angle of my head and my bulging neck veins.

"What is that?" he asked me, then turned to the midwives.

They leaned in, looked at it briefly, and ran their fingers over it. "Not sure, but you're doing great, Chantal. Keep breathing deeply and we'll look at it tomorrow."

"It's probably just a swollen pregnancy gland or weird milk duct that's backed into my neck."

I balked. Other than the odd cold here and there, I had never been sick a day in my life. I had had the most amazing pregnancy, and I felt stronger than ever. The thought did not even cross my mind that the lump might be something to worry about. Besides, I was a vegetarian yoga teacher who knew the law of attraction, so how could it be anything bad?

Two hours and only fifteen minutes of pushing later, my baby was born.

My sister cried out, "It's a boy!" as one of the midwives laid him on my chest for our first skin-to-skin, eye-to-eye-gaze, eternal bonding moment. I was exhilarated and completely in love. We all cried. He was perfect; the way he came into the world was perfect. In that moment, only perfection existed. I was totally in awe of what had just happened, at what my body knew to do. I had never had such an out-of-body experience while being so embodied at the same time. In the midst of birthing a human, I felt like the most wildly passionate and powerful goddess, a high priestess of life. With every breath, my body was the vessel bringing spirit into matter. In that life-altering moment, I was initiated by the Great Mother into Motherhood.

The day my son was born was one of the most joyful and celebratory high points in my life. It was also the same day a part of me died. Like a big exhale after the culmination of an inhale, following the climax of giving birth, there was a huge release. Through the portal of birth, I would come to face my own death. Indeed someone new was being born, but it wasn't only my child. It was the rebirth of my soul. In becoming a mother, I would come to discover that there truly is life after death.

Death

Three days later, upon the insistence of my midwives and my husband, I forced myself to go to the hospital, to have the lump near my collarbone looked at. It was December 21, winter solstice, also known as mid-winter, the longest night of the year. Although seasonally in nature it is a time predominated by darkness, winter solstice is also the very day when the light starts to wax and grow again. Symbolically, the darkest day of the year is also the day that marks the return of the light; the rebirth of the sun. Paradoxically, as the light was growing outwardly in the

Chapter One

world, inwardly, I was only beginning my journey into darkness.

Up until then, I had done everything I could to avoid going to a hospital for delivery; something about the clinical corridors and sterilizing fluorescent lights made me feel like pregnancy and childbirth were diseases to be cured and treated. Hospitals are where sick people go, I thought, and where people go to die. You can't help thinking about your own mortality when surrounded by sick and dying people. It was not exactly what I wanted to contemplate only days after giving birth.

When I resentfully arrived at the hospital, I remember feeling as though I was wasting my time. I really didn't think there was anything to be concerned about. I went to have the lump looked at, to put everyone else's mind at ease.

My first appointment was an ultrasound. When the ultrasound technician couldn't see the bottom of the lump on her screen, as it seemed to keep going below my collarbone, she sent me for an x-ray. I was then rushed to an emergency visit with the ear, nose, and throat specialist, and then off to get a biopsy, all within the span of three hours.

"What's with these people?" I wondered. "Why do they keep rushing me from one department to the next?" I barely had time to remove the sick gown in radiology when the nurse paged me up to the third floor for a biopsy.

I tried to convince myself that the overly burdened medical system was merely expediting the whole testing process because Christmas was three days away and they must have known I had a three-day-old baby at home, waiting to be breastfed. But as the sombre looks dawned on the faces of each of the medical technicians I saw, the idea that something might be wrong was becoming more of a possibility.

By this point, it was obvious that the lump was a swollen lymph node. Still unaware that this was anything to be concerned about, I asked the ENT specialist what swollen lymph nodes could

mean. My heart dropped when he gravely said, "Lymphoma."
"What the fuck? Isn't that cancer?" I recoiled.
"Yes. It could also be a symptom of cat scratch fever.... Have you been around any cats lately?" he asked in all seriousness.
"No, I hate cats," I cringed.
I don't really, but in that moment, I did. I had not been near any cats so I knew that was not what it was. But there was no way I could have cancer either. I was twenty-eight years old and healthy, I was a vegetarian yoga teacher, and I loved my life. I was happy and I had just had a baby! This was supposed to be the happiest time of my life, my full moon time to shine and celebrate. I believed cancer only happens to old people who smoke and eat junk food and think negative thoughts.

What was going on? Was this some weird postpartum nightmare I couldn't find my way out of? I wanted to wake up. I wanted all of it to go away. This wasn't supposed to be happening. My life had suddenly taken a turn and I didn't like where it was going.

"We'll have to wait until the biopsy results come back before we know anything for certain," the specialist tried to reassure me and himself. "In the meantime," he concluded, walking out of the examining room and sending me on my way, "enjoy the holidays with your family and new baby."

The cancer word, the c-bomb, had been dropped. I couldn't get it out of my mind. Waiting for the test results was even worse than getting the tests done. My husband and I tried to enjoy the holidays, our new little baby boy, and even my sister's engagement, which happened that Christmas Eve. But every night I sobbed, crying myself to sleep, fearing the worst.

"It's just your hormones, honey; everything's going to be fine," my mom would lovingly assure me.

"Seriously, Chant, you're the healthiest person I know. Just forget about it; it's probably a virus and your body is reacting

Chapter One

strangely because of the pregnancy." That is what everybody thought, and what we all wanted to believe.

The Call

Ten days later, on New Year's Eve, we got the call. I was sitting in the rocking chair, breastfeeding Ben in a momentary bubble of bliss, when the phone rang. Greg answered the call and went into our bedroom. I could hear him explaining, in a muffled voice, why I couldn't talk on the phone—I was busy feeding our newborn baby. "Mmhm ... yes doctor ... I understand ...." His voice sounded eerily stoic.

It was all taking too long. I was anxious to hear the news. I finished feeding Ben, handed him to mom, who was visiting for the first holidays with her first grandson, and joined Greg in our bedroom. We sat on the edge of the bed as he finished talking to the doctor. He ended the call and took my hand.

"SO ... what did he say?" I eagerly inquired.

"It was the ENT specialist calling from his ski holiday in Whistler," Greg answered.

"So...? And? What do I have?" I interrupted.

"He found out the test results as early as he could and wanted to give us the news personally. He even called us on his personal days off to let us know what was happening ... " Greg continued.

"And???" I urged him on.

"The results are not benign," he replied.

"What does that mean?"

"Chant, you have cancer."

Fear flooded my body, filling my veins like cold ice. White noise rang in my ears. Time stopped. My heart dropped, smashed to pieces on the floor. I felt the momentum of my life stop, like a Mack Truck crashing into a brick wall. The weird post-pregnancy nightmare was actually happening.

Wildfire Within

It was New Year's Eve, December 31, 2011. The Mayans had prophesied that the world would end in 2012, and, for me, it was proving to be true. Two thousand twelve was already shaping up to be the worst year of my life. Goodbye 2011, hello two thousand fucking twelve. I was watching all of the apocalyptic predictions happen before my very eyes. It was the end of the world. All of my well-laid plans and hopes and dreams vanished in an instant. This was it. I had cancer now; the good life was over. But, there was also a new child in our family and a new year was beginning. New life and death were happening all around me at the same time; I couldn't separate the two. Life turned into death, which turned into new life, like an endless wheel. I couldn't tell where life ended and death began, or where the past ended and the future began.

All I knew was that things would never be the same. My life went up in flames that day. Everything I had imagined for myself vanished with a phone call, devoured by the diagnosis. Disoriented by the turn of events, I felt myself inwardly spiralling out of control, confused, and unable to see clearly. When I tried to breathe deeply, sorrow clouded my lungs and tears flooded my eyes. Unable to feel the ground beneath my feet, I tried to find my bearings in the midst of a rapidly spreading wildfire.

Meditation and Medication

"We must be willing to let go of the life we have planned, so as to have the life that is waiting for us." Joseph Campbell

After the initial shock of receiving the diagnosis, we were catapulted into the all-too-frightening world of cancer. Further testing revealed that I had stage II Hodgkin's Lymphoma.

It was early January, and the doctors wanted me to start chemotherapy right away. Having seen my own grandmother

Chapter One

pass away from colon cancer in a hospital a decade earlier, I feared conventional medicine and didn't believe it to be an effective pathway to healing. I thought that the Western Medical model is partial and ineffective—doctors only treat symptoms, not the root of diseases, and they don't treat the individual as a holistic being. So when it came time to research treatment methods, naturally I looked for other options.

The worst thing to do, upon receiving any diagnosis, never mind a life-threatening one, is to google it. Avoid entering your disease into a search engine, at all costs. Yes, it's important to be informed and learn about the illness. But the internet is filled with so much information and so many horror stories that you'll drown out the only voice that really matters: the voice of your intuition. And this is the voice you most need to hear in times of crisis. No matter how many people have faced similar challenges, statistics and prognoses fail to capture the whole story. Odds of survival and chances of recovery are not one-size-fits-all. You are the only YOU there is and ever was. No matter how hard you try to follow someone else's road to recovery, you must claim responsibility for your own healing, and wildcraft your own path.

One of the comforting things I discovered, however, whilst researching and deciding what course of treatment to take, was the recurring theme of the power of belief. Bernie Siegel, MD (author of *Love, Medicine and Miracles*) and Bruce Lipton, PhD (author of *Biology of Belief*) speak in depth of a new biology. Drawing from the latest research in epigenetics and neuroscience, they describe how our belief about a treatment's efficacy can determine the outcome, and ultimately change the course of our life. Studies revealed that patients who did treatments with high hopes of recovery did better and recovered faster than their counterparts who feared or, even worse, didn't believe their treatments would work. It didn't matter what the treatment was; success rates were higher for those who believed their treatments would be successful, no matter what those treatments were.

Another pioneer researcher in this emerging biology of belief is Harvard medical graduate Kelly Turner, PhD, who authored *Radical Remission: Surviving Cancer Against All Odds*. Dr. Turner was fascinated by the fact that, although huge amounts of research had been done on the survival rates of cancer patients, no one had studied the thousands of people who had experienced radical remissions and healed from cancer. She coined the term "radical remission" instead of spontaneous remission, because she discovered there was nothing spontaneous about the cancer thrivers she was meeting. Instead, she studied what changes the survivors made, and found there were common lifestyle habits they all shared that led to their healing. Among these life changes were more outward lifestyle habits such as changing their diet and taking herbs, but the majority of the keys to healing in her findings were more inward in nature, such as following intuition, deepening a spiritual connection, and having strong reasons for living.

What I quickly discovered while exploring treatment options was that looking at statistics regarding survival rates was not the best use of my time. After doing so, I would usually end up sobbing on the floor, fearing that I might only have a few years left to live. I made the mistake, only once, of googling "Hodgkin's Lymphoma." Greg walked into the living room, only to see me curled in the fetal position crying on the floor at the thought that I might die before reaching the age of thirty.

"Let's make a deal," he said. "From now on, no more internet searches." He made me promise.

From that day onward, I never looked at anything cancer-related online again. I didn't want other people's negative stories to affect my belief about what lay ahead of me. My mind

Chapter One

was too sensitive and easily "imprintable." Reading about poor prognoses and random statistics only made me feel powerless and doomed to a destiny I did not like. As well-researched as the data may have been, statistics didn't (they simply can't) measure the full picture of what those studied people were doing behind the scenes to promote or halt their healing. And no matter what I read about my condition on the internet, I kept hearing a voice in my heart saying, "You are not a statistic! Choose a different outcome."

When faced with a spiritual health crisis, do not rely on the all-knowing Google-ji to predict your future. You have more effective things to do with your precious time, like meditating, praying, and reading inspiring stories about people who survived against all odds. Your cells are always listening to you, waiting to respond to your expectations. Instead of inhaling partial information from the internet or feeding off other people's fear-based reactions, fill your mind and heart with inspiring stories and teachings that will remind you of who you are and of what matters most.

As my husband and I explored all the treatment options, we prolonged making a decision for a few weeks. During that time, in between crying spells of despair and caring for a newborn baby, I read as many books as I could to explore alternative options.

Naturally, as a health-conscious yogi on my quest for treatments, I sought the counsel of a naturopath. A flight attendant-turned-naturopath friend of mine in Toronto advised me to look for a FABNO (Fellow of the American Board of Naturopathic Oncology) ND. With high hopes of being told that I could beat this thing with a few more greens and more positive thinking, I found Dr. Lemmo, an ND who specializes in oncology in Vancouver, and I booked an appointment right away.

Wildfire Within

When I went into his office a week later, I was mortified to see obituaries of past patients on a memo board in the waiting room. (Another what-not-to-do with someone newly diagnosed with cancer is to share stories of all the people who have died from it.)

As I looked around, surrounded by sickly looking elders frail from treatments, I was in disbelief that suddenly now, I too was a cancer patient. This was not supposed to be happening to me. What kind of negative vibrations or bad karma had got me into this nightmare? What had happened to my glamorous life of jet-setting and wine tastings and photo shoots? This couldn't be happening—there was some sort of cosmic mistake. I was too young and healthy, and I was happy, damn it! I loved my life before all this. And now, I was a mother. It wasn't even just about me anymore.

On the days when the "Why me?" bubble of despair would consume me, I would collapse in a crying heap on our bed. I'd sob for a while, then Greg would wrap Ben in a blanket, carry him into our room, and place him next to me. My baby looked adorable.

"Here's someone who'll make you feel better," Greg would say to try to comfort me.

Every ounce of me wanted to push them both away. I didn't want my baby to feel my sorrow or pick up on my pain. I wanted to protect him from knowing what was happening around him. "What did this precious little innocent being do to deserve a dying mother?" I'd wonder enraged.

Anger was something I experienced a lot throughout those early days of my diagnosis. But I was raised to be a good catholic girl. I strived to be a masterful yogini, and I was a people pleaser. If anger was there, I thought the most loving thing to do was pretend it wasn't, and hope it would go away. Anger was a negative emotion, I thought, a feeling I

Chapter One

did not want to feel. I thought I could positively think myself out of it. So, I would stuff it down and try to stifle the tears, long enough that eventually Benjamin's smile or warm scent would intoxicate me into forgetting what was really going on.

Meeting Dr. Lemmo, the ND FABNO, was a mildly entertaining encounter. He wore a gold chain under the collar of his shirt, didn't don the traditional white coat that doctors wear, and spoke with a mild Italian accent.

"Is this guy a real doctor?" Greg and I joked after leaving his office.

When we met with him the first time, I eagerly asked him what I could do to treat Hodgkin's naturally. I was convinced that I didn't want to do conventional chemotherapy, and I wanted to breastfeed my son for as long as I could. Dr. Lemmo proceeded to tell me that he rarely saw patients with Hodgkin's Lymphoma, because of the high success rate of conventional treatments. He recommended going through with the prescribed six rounds of chemotherapy to get rid of the cancer sooner, and in the meantime, we would keep my system fortified with intravenous vitamin C infusions.

"We can work on strengthening you during and after your treatments, but get it all over with sooner so you can move on with your life," he advised.

Although Dr. Lemmo was quirky, he was widely respected in his field. He was relaxed and relatable, and spoke to my human side that often felt ignored in the conventional medical rooms I came to know so well during that time. Intuitively, I trusted Dr. Lemmo.

After taking some time to cry, pray, read, reflect, and feel into what I felt would be the best course of action, I took his advice and decided to go through with chemotherapy.

One of the most sobering moments of receiving a cancer diagnosis is when you realize that you must go through it all alone. Most of your friends and family will be there to support you every step of the way but, in the end, you are the only one who can go through it. And go through it you must, like the infamous firewalkers of India who walk across burning embers. Life will give us many opportunities to move through discomfort. But, as in the traditional fire-walking ceremonies, these moments are not intended to harm us. They are uniquely calibrated for our soul's journey, brought forth to wake us up, fortify our spirit, and remind us of what lies within. Times of crisis and intensity can be devastating. But they can also be rites of passage, opportunities to embody courage, and invitations to stretch ourself into the person we long to be.

"Focus on what's possible, and what's possible will expand," my friend Christine Price Clark so eloquently once said. When faced with difficulties, we always have a choice to create more pain and separation by running away from the source of our discomfort, or we can turn toward the pain and learn to widen our embrace. Increase your faith in the potential for healing and more healing will occur. The sooner you realize that no one can walk over the burning embers for you, the more empowered you will be to choose how you're going to walk through those initiation portals. You must go through it, there is no choice there, but, as is true of any situation, you can always choose *how* you are going to go through it.

No matter how supported I was by friends and family, I was the only one who could create healing within myself. I had to take responsibility for my experience, and become the author of my life. Although at times I felt out of control and powerless, between the breakdowns I had momentary glimpses of my true nature. I knew intuitively, and from all my years of studying tantra and yoga, that although my body was experiencing disease, my spirit was still free, here to co-create with life.

The yogic teachings I have come to love have taught me that

Chapter One

everything is sacred and that, ultimately, we are here to grow our soul. In every moment, we are given the choice to evolve and expand. The tantric yogis believed that everything in life can become a blessing, and that the whole world is made of Divine Source Energy (they call it *Shiva* or *Shakti*, depending on their tradition). *Shiva* means "ground of being," "the medium of existence"; as in the air we breathe, the earth we walk upon, and consciousness itself. It also means "auspicious," "favourable," and "conducive to success." Success as described by the ancient yogis is not dependent on our financial status or Facebook following. Seeing life as a manifestation of Shiva is seeing the blessing in everything. It is recognizing that within each moment is a great gift. *Shakti* is the creative power of the Universe. Attuning to Shakti is sensing the vibratory possibility that exists within every breath. Put differently, from the tantric yogic perspective, everything is designed to evolve us.

I couldn't control what was happening around me, but I could choose how to walk through the fire. I couldn't change the fact that I had cancer, but I could choose how to respond to the changing winds. Instead of being the powerless victim, drifting in the unknown with no agency to affect my fate, when the wind did not blow my way, I could adjust my sails.

After consulting numerous other naturopaths, what felt like the best right path was to do the conventional treatments of chemotherapy and keep myself strong through high doses of vitamin C intravenously. As Dr. Lemmo advised, I could focus on fortifying my body during chemotherapy and work to restore and rejuvenate myself after the treatments were over. I reasoned that we could spend time trying to cure the cancer naturally, without conventional chemotherapy, but if the less-invasive natural methods weren't effective, we'd risk having to do the harsher treatments later on. And by then, my son would be crawling or walking.

"Do the treatments now, while he's too young to remember what's happening, and move on with your life," I was told by all the doctors, and more importantly, by my intuition.

I was heartbroken. My whole sense of identity as a healthy, positive, globe-trotting yogi was shattered, burned away, and destroyed. I believed in the power of nature so deeply, yet not enough that I would choose to heal myself without conventional medicine. Suddenly I felt like a fake, a failure, and a hypocrite. My ego was crushed, and it was excruciating. But the most painful part was trying to hold onto the life I had once known. My grip on how I thought life should be was so tight. I was spending so much energy clenching onto what I wanted, pushing against what was happening, wishing it would be different, that I exhausted myself. As the sleepless nights of stress and tending to our new baby accumulated, I knew I needed to muster all the energy I could to make it through this. I could keep wasting my precious life force energy trying to resist the death my familiar self was experiencing, or I could drop the struggle and open to where life was taking me.

With a deep exhale, I released the resistance to what was.

Perhaps, this crucible was an initiation, I thought to myself. Could it be that the pain I was feeling was a growing pain, the discomfort of being stretched beyond what I had known before? Maybe I was being cleansed on a deep soul level, to be strengthened and vivified. Trial by fire, a burning away of all that I was not, so I could become all that I truly am. I had given birth only a few weeks earlier to another human. Now, I had to give birth all over again. This time, to my true self.

Contraction and Expansion

"Spiritual growth is like childbirth. You dilate, then you contract. You dilate, then you contract again. As painful as it all feels,

Chapter One

it's the necessary rhythm for reaching the ultimate goal of total openness." Marianne Williamson, *A Woman's Worth*

When a woman gives birth, she physically shifts from maidenhood—the fertile innocent time of budding potential—into motherhood—the blooming season of giving life and taking care of others. To be a great mother, whether of a child or a creative project, a woman must also learn to nurture herself. Transition times, when we're leaving something behind, yet not fully embodying who we're growing into, are uncomfortable and often made more painful by our resistance to them.

I wanted the cancer to go away as quickly as possible, so I could move on with my life. I found my entire being resisting having to go through any of it—resisting accepting what my life had become, resisting the prescribed course of action, resisting my own feelings of resistance. I was resisting and pushing against the necessary contractions that precede any expansion.

Having just gone through the most empowering birth experience weeks before, the physical sensation of giving birth was still imprinted in my body. One thing I had learned from giving birth to my own son and through all my prenatal studies was that fear slows labour. Fear shifts us into fight-or-flight mode, and pulls our attention and energy from the task at hand (giving birth) to sending vital blood supply to other body parts. If a woman is fearful of birth, her labour slows (even stops) and she is deemed as "failing to progress."

This feature of our psychosomatic physiology has been a necessary part of our survival; if a woman were giving birth in the wild and a tiger appeared, the cervix would contract tightly to halt the labour, until she could move to a safe place to birth her baby. And thank goodness for that. It makes sense that real progress in any endeavour cannot happen when we are fearful.

Wildfire Within

In the presence of fear, we contract for protection; we close down. Fear stems from an evolutionary impulse to survive, and it is beneficial at times. In her book *Big Magic*, Elizabeth Gilbert highlights that fear has kept us alive as a species. We would not have survived without it. Fear can be a healthy response to things unknown, yet we don't want to live in a state of fear, in a constant state of contraction, always closing ourselves off to what wants to come through us. Perhaps it is true that we've survived as a species because of fear. But as humans we've thrived and flourished because of our creativity and our ability to dream something new into being. Although labouring women no longer have to run from real tigers in the wild, metaphorical tigers still show up as the stressors of our daily life. We are not meant to live in fear. It keeps us closed, and running from tigers that are not really there.

There is a difference between contracting and closing. Contracting is the necessary precursor to expanding; it has focus and intent. It's a loving squeeze from the Universe, my teacher Sianna says. Closing because of fear is what keeps expanding from happening; fear closes our hearts and constricts our body's intelligence. We are wired to survive, and fear is a protective mechanism with an agenda to preserve and keep things the same. You could say fear blocks our innate evolutionary impulse to expand, and that's why it's so paralyzing and painful when we find ourselves inundated with it.

In the process of giving birth, there exists a fear-tension-pain cycle. When we're fearful, our muscles contract and tense up in preparation to fight or take flight, which creates a more painful labour, because it's going against what the body naturally wants to do: to open. The most effective antidote is to accept and trust the process (a woman's body knows how to birth a baby), relax, and even try to enjoy the experience. "Progress" and enjoyment in labour can happen when a woman consciously relaxes, lets

Chapter One

go of the tension, and releases the resistance. In the same way, fear slows labour and delays the blossoming of our soul. It keeps us locked into habitual ways of being, closing us off from the beauty of life. Evolution and magic happen when you trust the process, and ride the momentum of where life wants to take you.

One of the biggest tragedies of receiving a cancer diagnosis is that it is an event marked by so much fear that we become paralyzed by it. What an immense opportunity it could be, to wake up to the beautiful fragility of life, to cherish the gift of our embodiment. Instead, fear floods our system and we begin to attack the very body in which we live with our thoughts and fears and treatments. We silence the wisdom and innate intelligence of our immune system and start to fight against it, instead of learning how to listen and support it.

How much more effective could treatments and healing modalities be, I wonder, if we could approach the whole topic with less of a fearful charge? Not only do we have to deal head on with fear of our own mortality when newly diagnosed, but we also have to manage everyone else's fears too. Of course it is only natural to become fearful when faced with the potential of our death. But guess what? It's going to happen eventually, to everyone. Cancer simply forces us to get clear about what really matters, and decide how we want to spend our limited time here on earth.

The number of times I had to console my friends when I told them I had cancer was exhausting. "You're going to be okay right?" they would naturally worry.

"Yes, of course, don't worry about me," I would assure them, then do everything in my power to protect them from the pain and inevitability of them facing their mortality, as a result of me being faced with mine.

I read once that what you're most afraid of has already

happened. In my case, the death of my ego, my self-identity, had already occurred. I was afraid of dying, and in a way, when I was told I had cancer, the me I thought I was died. Although my body was still physically alive, my sense of self was shattered.

In childbirth, all we need to "do" is relax, and trust that our body knows how to birth a baby. Fear and tension only prolong and inhibit the process. During labour, the more we trust and relax, the more the body will open and attune to its innate capacity to expand. When birthing a human and while going through any major life transition, true power lies in releasing resistance. One of my teachers, Hareesh (Christopher Wallis), says that whenever we resist what life is offering us, we suffer. When we accept how life wants to shape us, everything unfolds for our benefit. The yogis recognize that there is great power in relaxation; there is power in letting go.

In receiving a cancer diagnosis, I came face to face with the fact that I would die, perhaps sooner than I wanted. But in the same breath, I was given a chance to rebirth myself. I could become my own midwife, and bring forth the person I wanted to be. Midwives never take the credit for delivering the baby, they simply let nature do its thing, and are there to catch the baby. In the same way, we cannot force our way through our challenges or simply push through the pain. We can't rush birth, and we can't rush growth. Like gestating a human or planting a seed, the blooming process has its own timing. We can't rush it, nor can we stop it from happening. All we can do is be present to it, witness the process, and attune to where we are along the creative process, our soul's journey, so we can do what is required with the most grace and ease. In becoming our own midwives, we become willing participants in our own unfolding.

Chapter One

Pulse and Flow

The natural expansion and contraction of childbirth can be witnessed in nature by observing the cycles of the moon. Every month, the moon's light waxes, growing toward fullness (expansion), then wanes and recedes back to darkness (contraction). Pulsing between waxing and waning, the moon follows a rhythm, and it is this vital rhythm that allows life to flourish. With its peak culmination of light and effulgent radiance, the full moon is symbolic of giving birth, and the peak point where energy begins to recede once more.

The tantric yogis understood that there is a great pulsation at the heart of the Universe that creates the rhythm of life. This sacred throb or holy vibration is found throughout all of creation. In Sanskrit, they call it *spanda*, the recognition that everything in the Universe is vibrating and always pulsing between expansion and contraction. Through allurement, stars contract energy into their centre, then expand with light. The moon appears to wax and wane, ocean waves rise and fall with the ever-ebbing and flowing tides. Our heart beats, our lungs expand and contract with every breath; orgasms and childbirth are full of *spanda*. Everything is pulsating with this eternal breath of creation, the living heartbeat of the Universe.

As a culture, we tend to favour the expansion part. We love the moreness of life, and are always seeking to grow. But we forget that we cannot experience expansion without seasons of contraction. We don't value the necessary release process that must come before any further expansion. In fact, we put a lot of effort into avoiding contractions, or times of apparent loss and simplification. But if we are willing to really ride the wave, embrace the fullness of being human, and allow the necessary contractions of life to occur, then we open ourselves to the greater expansion that always, inevitably follows. If we resist the contractions, labour becomes painful and development is arrested as we fight against our own growth. We "fail to progress."

The more we can align with nature's wild yet wise rhythms and waves of pulsing energy, the more we can harness the inherent power of the current, live with more ease and flow, and experience deeper wellbeing. For it is only in the descent, in the moving through the dark and deep mysterious phases of our soul's journey, that we can truly rise up and come to know who we really are. It is only by giving way to the contractions, that we can truly expand. The full moon can only be made new again, by turning toward the dark.

CHAPTER TWO

Flames: You Will Find a Way (Disseminating Moon)

Disseminating Moon: Gather, relax, accept, understand, regroup, wander

"'I'm an adventurer, looking for treasure.'" Paulo Coelho, *The Alchemist*

The Disseminating Moon

After the moon's light reaches its peak with the full moon, it begins its journey back toward darkness via the disseminating moon. The word *disseminate* means "to distribute or scatter about," as in, "to sow seeds." Here the moon carries the energy of gathering new insights as she surrenders back into the mystery of the unknown. It is the first phase of the waning process, when it seems like everything we have known is falling apart. Energetically, it isn't the time to start something new, but to be gentle with ourself and regroup our forces.

Like the cycles of the moon, throughout the adventure of our life, we are always moving through phases; away from one thing and toward another. Life, as we know it, ends and begins again many times within the course of our one life. There are many jumping off points—moments when we depart from what we have known, and live into the mysterious space between what has been, and what is yet to come. The first time we leave home (the familiar world we have known) and experience transition (get the job, move to another city, receive a diagnosis) are such departure moments.

Some transitions are easier than others. And then there are those disseminating pivot points that will change the trajectory of our life forever, when the clarity we have known is replaced with uncertainty, and our comfortable way of being in the world no longer works for what is being asked and required of us.

The Space Between

Amidst the moon's phases and on the soul's journey, the in-between place is often described as the underworld. The space between is the descent into the unfamiliar places within, of shadow and the not-yet discovered. The moon's trajectory and the soul's journey are not upward linear roads from A to B. The moon moves in cycles. The way of the soul is circuitous, having many twists and turns and perfectly timed detours along the way. We have to be willing to journey into the mysterious and fertile unknown that is like the moon's dark side, before we can rise up radiant, rooted into who we really are.

We leave our familiar life as we've known it, and journey down into the dark night to discover parts of ourselves we have not yet known. We undergo a naked encounter with the heart of who we really are, the unique soul essence we are here to embody. Ultimately, no one can avoid journeying into the underworld, from those dark times in life, as high as we might try to jump over them. But if we learn to trust the spanda, the natural pulsation of life, then we can emerge from the underworld forever changed and transformed, bringing with us lessons learned, which

Chapter Two

become our gifts and medicine for ourselves and our people. If we dare journey into the deep questions and dark emotional crevices of our experience, we always return expanded.

When leaving on any journey, it's always helpful to know the destination. Where you want to go will determine what you pack and how you plan to get there. On the quest of living into your soul's purpose, there is an intuitive nudge, a dream in your heart, like a deep root system within that governs all of your choices. Learning to trust your desires and follow your inner knowing is essential to navigating the dark night when it seems as though everything is falling apart. Listening to your intuition will always light the way.

Yet, no matter how well prepared you are, the adventure of your life cannot be predicted or experienced by setting goals, studying a map, or by simply deciding where you want to end up. Like the soul's journey, the road to fulfillment is not a one-way ticket to some better place, but rather a living, dynamic journey that is meant to grow and evolve you. The destination on the soul's journey is not a physical place, but a way of being in your own heart, body, and life. To experience the enriching journey itself is the goal, the means by which you learn to embody your soul and live to know deeper levels of joy and freedom. The soul's journey is not about filling a void or reaching an external destination at some future point in time, but rather it is like questing for the Holy Grail, and discovering that the Holy Grail is inside you. It is not about filling yourself up with something from outside yourself, but a movement of bringing forth what is within you, into the living expression of your life.

Our culture has taught us to look outside ourselves for answers and fulfillment. We are told that all we need to do is work harder and buy bigger and better things to fill the emptiness we feel inside. But the clarity and contentment we seek is not something we can chase, earn, or acquire, like the latest fashion we can buy at the store. Experiencing deep joy is rather a by-product, a welcomed side effect of soulful living. The inner peace we all long for does not come from the adornments we don, but from consciously tending to the inner fire we each carry. The fire in the heart is the presence of soul, the unique expression of the Divine through us, as us. And like a living fire, the soul flame within needs kindling and oxygen to stay alive and vital. When the road is dark, that is when we must turn inward and fan the flame the most, and trust that the vision we carry within ourselves—of the life we long to live while we're here—will light the way to who we're here to become.

Fanning the fire in your heart is not something to add to the bottom of your to-do list, nor is it the thing you'll get to once you've checked off all your other tasks. Soulful living is not something that will just happen later on, when you finally have some free time for "self-care." It doesn't come from reading self-help books or attending weekend workshops. Fanning the flame is a daily remembrance that you are here to grow. It's about choosing to nourish what is most important first. The journey of becoming who we're meant to be in this world requires dedication, consistency, and courage; yet keeping the inner fire lit, especially when the road seems dark, is the most vital work we can do with our life force.

View from the Top

My first big departure, my journey into the unknown, was when I left home to work for the airline at nineteen years of age. My father, an airline pilot, encouraged me to apply for a summer job as a flight attendant when he heard his employer was hiring. Dad loved everything about aviation. He had model airplanes of the entire Air Canada fleet in our basement rec room, and he framed old aviation calendars, hung them around our home, and called them art.

Chapter Two

At the time, I was waiting tables at Joey Tomato's in Calgary, not quite sure what I wanted to do with my life. I was taking courses in business, philosophy, anatomy, and interior design at Mount Royal University. These were all things I was interested in, but I was not really sure how I could stitch them together into any sort of cohesive career.

Dad and I flew to Toronto for my first Air Canada flight attendant interview. Thousands of people were there from all over the country. When we arrived, it looked like an audition for *American Idol* with a sea of talented candidates lining the corridor of the Westin Harbour Castle Hotel. I was nervous, but figured all I could do was be myself, and highlight that I was bilingual in English and French.

"And don't forget to mention your dad is a pilot," Dad reminded me, as he dropped me off in front of the hotel.

Three interviews, two personality tests, and a language proficiency exam later, I was offered the job. Hired as a flight attendant for the summer, I was sent to Montreal for initial training. For the first time, I left the comfort of my parents' home and tasted freedom. Liberated from the suburban nest of my upbringing, my eyes opened to the vastness of opportunity that exists when we take a leap into the unknown.

During initial flight attendant training, we practised evacuation drills by day, and danced in the bars of Le Plateau by night. I fell in love with the culture, the old buildings, and the creative energy of Montreal. *Le Vieux-Montréal* reminded me of my first trip to Paris the year before. I fed off the electric pulse of the city and realized how much I love to speak French. My sensual and romantic inner self comes to life when I speak it. Life's melodramas become more poetic and beautiful somehow; and I feel more feminine when I speak my mother tongue, which I had learned before I learned English, having been born and raised the first few years of my life in St-Boniface, a French-speaking community in Manitoba.

For the first time, I could imagine a bigger more interesting life outside the familiar suburban life I had experienced in Calgary up until then. My boyfriend of the time, Ashton, was not thrilled about my newfound freedom as a flight attendant. He resented the fact that I was gone so much, and didn't like how distracted I was by my new friends and adventurous trips. At the time, I was still very much in love with him and still very concerned about pleasing other people, so I planned to move back to Calgary as soon as I could, to keep him happy and resume our relationship.

After training ended, we new flight attendants kissed Montreal au revoir, and went to Air Canada's Toronto base to crew all the busy summer flights. As it was only a temporary summer job and knowing that I had no intention of putting down roots in Toronto, I joined a dozen of my new commuter friends, and moved into a crash pad on Dixon Road, a few blocks away from the airport. There were twelve of us in a three-bedroom apartment, four air mattresses to each room. Oh, the glamour!

On the rare occasion that more than four of us would be at the apartment at the same time, we'd invite other out-of-town commuters from buildings in the neighbourhood over for dinner, and have wine and dance parties in the living room. Being the newest and most junior flight attendants (FAs), we were all at the bottom of the seniority list and on reserve. We were the backup crew when the more senior FAs would book time off or take summer vacation. In those first summer months on call, we could end up anywhere in the world with only an hour's notice.

At the entrance of our temporary crash pad home, we hung a large whiteboard on the wall, and there we'd write the place we'd been sent to, to let our roommates know where we were

Chapter Two

and when we'd be back. "Gone to Santiago, back on Thursday, Sebastian." "Max in HKG." "Ingrid in Delhi!" "Valerie, Paris." "Sophie, Tokyo." "Sylvain, Winnipeg."

Spreading my newfound wings that summer, I was invigorated by the expanded perspective that travelling allows. I tasted the freedom that comes from being in a new environment every day, and fell deeply in love with the world. I went to London, Hong Kong, Tokyo, and New York. Frankfurt and Shanghai, Paris and Istanbul became my favourite shopping spots. I saw every major Canadian city: Ottawa, Vancouver, Montreal; and some minor ones too: Deer Lake, St. John's, Regina.

From the top, the view was magnificent. The world became so small, yet so vast, and I wanted to experience it all.

Wandering into Yoga

Yoga had come into my life the year before, when I was eighteen. My grandmother had passed away of colon cancer, and I was by her side as she died. Seeing her transition from this life, I was faced with my own mortality for the first time, and realized in a visceral way that I too would have to let go of life one day. As a very young adult, this was not something I had given much thought to before. But being by my grandmother's side as she passed changed the course of my life. It catalyzed my spiritual search for meaning and purpose. Looking back now, I see how this was really the beginning of my quest as a seeker; it was such a gift.

Not long after she died, in search of spiritual solace, I went to my first yoga class at the Ashtanga Yoga Shala on Nineteenth Street in Calgary, with my boyfriend Ashton. He played basketball for the University of Calgary team at the time, and had heard that yoga would be good for his game, so he came along. Ashtanga Yoga is a particularly dynamic form of yoga that links breath with movement and emphasizes building strength, flexibility, and stamina through its set sequence in the Primary (and subsequent) Series. It is a very vigorous form of yoga and so appeals to the more athletic seekers.

It was love at first Downward-Facing Dog. Walking into the studio felt like coming home. The Yoga Shala—*shala* is a Sanskrit word referring to a sacred yoga space—was adorned with antique, dark wooden armoires and gorgeous golden fabrics from Mysore, India. The scent of Nag Champa Incense sweetened the air. Black and white pictures of yogis and wise sages hung on the walls. People passing through the yoga studio always seemed happier and healthier than those outside the studio walls. When I first began yoga, I was drawn to the embodied spirituality it offered. The simplicity of feeling my breath and moving my body in unison reminded me of how miraculous it is to be alive.

When I became a flight attendant, every time I visited a new city for more than twenty-four hours I looked for a yoga studio where I could unroll my mat. It became my lifeline to a sense of stability and grounding in my otherwise turbulent life. I knew I wanted to learn more about yoga and I inhaled all the books I could find on the subject.

Mother India

Naturally, being fascinated with yoga, I was thrilled one morning when I got a call from crew scheduling sending me to New Delhi. Most people loathed this flight. It was fifteen hours from Toronto with demanding and generally messy passengers. I had heard horror stories of really old people peeing or dying on their seat, and of babies being stored in overhead bins. But none of the stories swayed me. I was enchanted with the idea of going to Mother India, the birthplace of yoga and

Chapter Two

many of the world's major religions. I knew it held deep magic for me. It would be my first pilgrimage to a far and ancient land where I could meet a wise guru who would give me all the answers to my existential questions, and offer me a direct transmission of all the secrets to life.

"Miss, please, coke for my baby," a young Indian woman asked coyly in the back galley, five hours into the flight, a beige sari sliding off the side of her static, airplane hair. She held her three-month-old baby in one arm, and extended her other that was holding an empty bottle for me to fill.

"Coke?" I asked shocked that anyone would give her young baby coke. "No, Madame, I'll give you milk or water instead, but I won't give you coke for your baby."

Not fully understanding what I said, she handed over the bottle. I filled it with milk, placed it in a coffee carafe filled with boiling water to heat it, and watched it bobble there a few minutes before handing it back. She looked disappointed but didn't speak enough English to protest my intervention; she returned to her seat.

On a flight as long as the one to New Delhi from Toronto, the crew gets a four- to six-hour break to sleep in the crew bunks between services. I opted for the later break and rode my excitement out by staying up as long as I could. While half the crew went down into the underbelly bunks for the first break, I sat in the back row and pulled from my bag a newly purchased book I'd bought at the airport before boarding the flight to New Delhi. *The Alchemist* by Paulo Coelho had come highly recommended by my gorgeous French yogi roommate Sophie. She had a beautiful smile and a sparkle in her eyes. She claimed yoga saved her life after years of depression and suicidal urges. I never would have known she had once suffered so much inside, from seeing the glow she emitted now. I wanted what she had. I wanted to know the secrets she knew about the eradication of sorrow. So I read *The Alchemist* cover to cover in one sitting, during my four-hour break.

"No heart has ever suffered when it goes in search of its dreams, because every second of the search is a second's encounter with God and with eternity." Paulo Coelho, *The Alchemist*

I gleaned some gems from the book—choose to seek your destiny; craft your personal legend; follow your heart, and alchemize difficulties into gold. Reading *The Alchemist* was an energizing life-giving elixir, providing nourishing green juice to my thirsty soul.

When we landed in New Delhi, I looked out my jump seat window and saw a dog chasing a monkey down the runway before the golden setting sun. Like Dorothy waking up in the land of Oz, I knew I wasn't in Canada anymore!

As soon as they opened the aircraft door, the humid thickness of India filled the airplane. It smelled of distant burning fires, warmth, and sweetness. The density of the place was palpable. Even the air here felt ancient. I could feel the depth and richness of the land with each inhale that filled my lungs. I loved the spiritual heaviness of the atmosphere.

The drive to the hotel from the New Delhi airport was long. We drove through shanty towns of cardboard dwellings on the sides of the highway, into a ritzy part of Delhi where our crew hotel was located. We arrived at the gates of the Marriot Hotel to see a banner draped over the iron entryway, formally welcoming the President of Mexico, who was also staying at our hotel that night. Upon arrival, we checked into our rooms, sent our uniforms for dry cleaning with the hotel butler, freshened up, and met down in the international airline crew lounge for a drink before heading out for dinner.

In the lounge, there were crews from Australia, Germany, Thailand, and the UK. One of the young Indian girls from

Chapter Two

our crew spoke Hindi. She did this route weekly and visited her family during her layovers.

"I'm heading to a rave outside the city with my cousins; not sure what time I'll be back at the hotel or if I'll even make it back tonight. Want to come?"

As exciting and adventurous as the thought of going to a psychedelic dance party with thousands of people in a distant Indian jungle sounded, it was a little too wild and required more courage or stupidity than I had at the time. "I think I'll pass, but have fun," I answered.

"I'm going to the antique market tomorrow," another flight attendant named Irene chimed in. "There are beautiful saris and spices there too, if you want to join me."

"Yes!" I exclaimed. "That's exactly what I want to do while I'm in India for two days."

After dinner, I hit the pillow and slept like a baby until the next morning. As planned, I met some of my crew members in the lobby. After breakfast, we hopped in a taxi and headed to Sunder Nagar Market.

Driving in New Delhi is terrifying. At every turn and merge on the wide chaotic highway, I saw my short life flash before my very eyes. Eight lanes wide with no dividing lines, the roads are a crazy mess and it's a miracle anyone gets to where they're going in one piece. Rickshaws, tuk-tuks, and mopeds weave in between cars. Some scooters have entire families of five on board, with three kids hanging off the sides.

"HORN OK PLEASE" is painted boldly in bright yellow on the back of big green trucks. A cacophony of car horns, motors putting, and the hum of thousands of people fill the air, each person making their way to their destination; every moment on the road is a chaotic intersection of millions of destinies colliding.

"How does anyone get to where they're going?" I asked, laughing in amazement.

Wildfire Within

"Relax, miss, no one is in control," chuckled the driver, peering at me over his shoulder in the rearview mirror that was adorned with a little hanging Ganesha figurine.

A garland of marigolds hung along the inside of the taxi's windshield, and a little blue Krishna sticker danced on his dash. We came to a stop for a red light, and were immediately surrounded by a dozen young children, pouring their arms and grasping hands into the car, asking for rupees. "Please, miss. Rupee, please."

"Don't give them anything," murmured my fellow passengers, the four of us comfortably squished in the back seat. "They don't get to keep the money; it goes to their pimping beggar boss."

Heartbroken by the thought of these young children being enslaved, I threw some bills at them as the light turned green and we drove away.

The intense paradox of India is striking. Ornate palaces behind large iron gates are surrounded by fields of perfectly cut, lush green grass; crippled beggars and cardboard shacks; brightly coloured saris and handwoven fabrics; bold fuchsias, deep blues, golden oranges for miles. Stray dogs run into oncoming traffic. The scent of sweet spices infuses the air. Men squat, drinking Chai beside street food carts. The sounds of scooters, tuk-tuks, and mopeds buzz in the air. The electrical wires from all directions chaotically converge into a gigantic knotted bundle at the top of the telephone poles, sparks flying. There is so much beauty and so much suffering, all at the same time.

We survived the drive, somewhat stunned to have made it out alive, and arrived at the antique market before lunch. Shaped like a curved horseshoe, the market place is lined with tea shops, spice stands, and antique shops; gorgeous multicoloured saris hang from above, creating a multicoloured tapestry in the sky.

"The antique shop in the corner is the one you must check

Chapter Two

out. The shopkeeper reads palms. And he's always right." Irene pointed to a little hidden door beneath a canopy as she walked in the other direction toward her favourite teashop. "I'll meet you back here in half hour," she waved as she walked away.

I headed into the shop near the far end of the market. Walking through the doors was like entering a cave of wonders. Brass lamps, copper frames, Hindu *murtis*, and silver candle holders hung from every available wall and ceiling space. I found a set of tingsha bells, the small cymbals attached by a leather strap that yoga teachers use at the end of a class to awaken their students from Savasana, the final resting pose at the end of every class, and I made my way to the desk to pay.

Seated on a wooden stool behind the low desk, the shopkeeper wore a white turban and a burgundy button up, short sleeve shirt. He was younger than I had expected, but old enough that his short beard had patches of grey peppered throughout. I placed the bells on the heavy wooden desk as he looked up with a warm smile in his eyes. "Are you the one who reads palms?" I asked hesitantly.

"Yes, my dear, it is I. Have a seat, please. " He gestured his outstretched arm toward the stool across from him, nodding his head in a gentle up-and-down, side-to-side bobble.

I sat down and extended my open palm. He took it is his hand and examined it closely.

"Ah," he exclaimed. "You will have many riches in your life." My skepticism increased; it sounded like a line he started every session with. Furrowing his thick eyebrows, he continued. "And the one you are with now, he is not the one. It will end in infidelity. I am sorry, dear."

"Oh, okay, thank you." I withdrew my hand from his open palm and decided I had heard enough.

Although things had been rocky between Ashton and me, I still loved him and wasn't ready to call it quits. Somewhat annoyed at the shopkeeper's prediction, I left money for the tingsha bells and headed toward the door. But before I could leave the store, he got up and walked toward me, stopping in front of me, blocking my exit. Suddenly nervous that I had offended him, I looked up as he gently took my hand and placed a small metal figurine in my palm, closing my fingers over it with his other hand.

"Here, take this. She will help you. Pray to her and become the artist of your life. Life is the canvas, you are the painter."

I opened my closed fist to peer at what he had given me.

"Saraswati," he said. "Saraswati is the goddess of wisdom and creativity," he explained. She was sitting on a swan and holding a long-stringed instrument. I felt a surge of calm rush through me as I held her tightly, close to my heart.

"Thank you," I spoke, leaving the store, unsure of what had just happened.

I left feeling irritated; yet shifted. Something seemingly magical had occurred. I felt more awake and alive than I had before going into the store. Maybe I was just adjusting to the time zone. But the colours in the square looked more vivid. There was suddenly a calmness to all the chaos swirling around me.

Seeing the other crew members standing at the entrance of the market, I walked toward them to tell them all about the shopkeeper's predictions. As we stood on the corner sidewalk, suddenly a gorgeous elephant turned a corner, walking toward us. Pink, white, and yellow flowers and paint adorned his gentle face.

"Oh my god! That's amazing. Does this always happen?" I asked Irene in awe, with a grin from ear to ear.

"I do this pairing every month and have never seen an elephant in the city before!" she said. "This has never happened in the fifteen years I've been coming here."

Chapter Two

As the majestic creature approached us, his rider—his mahout—gave him a gentle tap behind his ear. The elephant knelt down in front of us as his rider signaled to Irene and me to climb on. Sensing the magic in the moment, a wink from the Universe nudging me on, I mounted the beautiful animal and straddled her wide back, sitting behind the rider. With a tap of the mahout's stick behind her ear, we strolled around the market, bystanders surrounding us on both sides, also in awe of a massive elephant walking through the crowded market. I couldn't believe my luck. I sat back and took in the amazement of being on an elephant's back in India. Just another day on the job, I thought, in pure appreciation of the richness of the moment.

Later we met up with the rest of the crew and our driver, and made our way back to the hotel. I went for a swim in the pool and an Ayurvedic oil massage at the hotel spa. When I returned to my room, my dry-cleaned uniform hung in the closet. Feeling rejuvenated, I slept soundly in the moonlight that poured through the palm trees, in through my window.

"Don't eat the street food; you'll get Delhi belly," everyone had warned me. I had heard that people experienced culture shock in India, and that my delicate Canadian digestion could not handle the bacteria in the water supply. But India was good for my system. Like an energy boost for my soul, it awakened my senses and opened me to the vast mystery of life. I did not experience culture shock in India; I experienced an awakening of magic.

The next morning we boarded our fifteen-hour flight back to Toronto. The flight home was smooth. Getting back to my apartment, I unpacked my suitcase and found the little Saraswati *murti* I had rolled up in a t-shirt. I placed her on my bookshelf next to a family picture and the few yoga books I had. I would visit India again, I decided. To go on a pilgrimage to the motherland of yoga, see the sacred sites, and look for a real yogi guru.

A few weeks later, things fell apart between Ashton and me. Since I started flying, he had felt quite lonely. As it turned out, he had met someone else.

You Will Find a Way

The only bug I caught in India was the travel bug. Ever since returning from New Delhi, I dreamed of going back to the motherland of yoga.

I bid for my vacation time, and immediately started looking for places to visit where I could learn about yoga and Ayurveda. With a low budget, I stumbled upon a website that placed seeking travellers in various Indian ashrams at a fraction of the cost of other retreats, in exchange for some *seva* ("selfless service" or "volunteer work"). One of the programs offered a two-week stay at an ashram in Goa, with some volunteer time at the local orphanage. It was exactly what I was looking for. I signed up right away and prepared for my return voyage to India.

After doing some online research, I discovered I would need a visa for my return visit. I could send my passport away by registered mail, and hope to have it returned within a few weeks with an Indian visa enclosed. Because I was a flight attendant and needed my passport to work and fly, I couldn't be without it for that long. I needed another option. Upon further reading, it appeared I could apply in person for an expedited twenty-four-hour visa process. The next day, I visited the Indian Consulate on Bloor Street in downtown Toronto.

When I got to the consulate, I was surprised to see how many other people also needed to speak to the Indian Consulate's staff. Apparently I wasn't the only special case. There were

Chapter Two

hundreds of people, most of them Indian, all there for different reasons, and all needing help from above.

With a melodic hum of Hindi and Punjabi ringing through the air, I stood in line with high hopes, for four hours. When I finally got to the desk, the consulate lady sweetly explained, "Sorry, I cannot help you, the expedited visa is for very special cases only. You need to speak to my superior."

Perfect, I thought, surely her boss would understand and appreciate that I was going to do some volunteer work and spend money in his country; he would help me out. I was given an appointment for two weeks later.

Enthused by the idea that my dream trip to India was closer to becoming a reality, I headed back to the Indian Consulate on the scheduled day. I arrived, waited a while, and was relieved when my name was finally called: "Miss Chantil, please come." A middle-aged Indian woman escorted me into the Consul General's office. I was being taken to see the top dog, the highest Indian authority in Canada.

Sitting across from the Consul General, I stated my case. "Thank you for meeting with me, sir. I'd like to go to India to volunteer in an orphanage and learn about yoga. I can't be without my passport for work. Can you please process my visa application in twenty-four hours, as I've heard you're able to do, sir?"

The tall man leaned back in his chair and shook his head from side to side with a slight up and down motion, which turned into the subtle bobble I had seen weeks earlier. Not sure if he was signaling yes or no, I waited with bated breath for his response.

With a thick Hindi accent, he finally answered. "I am sorry, dear. I cannot help you."

"What? What do you mean? Why not?" I explained again the nature of my profession and my plans to do good work in his country. Surely he would support my cause.

"The special twenty-four-hour processing is only available in emergencies. There is nothing I can do for you. I am so sorry," he concluded, leaning back in his chair, with his dark eyes set on mine, head still bobbling. His mind was made up.

"Well, if you can't help me get into the country, then who can? How will I get to India?" I anxiously asked.

He leaned forward in his chair, put his elbows on his desk and brought the tips of his long fingers together in prayer. Suddenly, he took on a sage-like demeanour, looked at me with his piercing brown eyes and replied in his thick Hindi accent, "You will find a way. You will find a way. You WILL find a way."

After a slight pause, he stood up from his chair and pointed toward to the door.

Stunned, defeated, and speechless, I left his office unsure of what to do next. How on earth would I find my way to India without a visa?

Totally discouraged and humbled, I wondered how I could make this trip happen. My vacation time was a month away. With no Indian visa, I'd have to cancel my volunteering ashram plans and go elsewhere. On the way home, it dawned on me that there really wasn't anything else I could do to get to India. Feeling disheartened, I wondered how I would ever become a real yogi without going to India. Riding the subway on the way home, I asked the Universe to let me know where she wanted me to go. Mother India was clearly sending me elsewhere; it was not yet time to go back. I had dreams, but I didn't know how to make them happen. Rather than trying to figure it all out, I opened myself to be led.

"You will find a way." The Consul General's response became a mantra, echoing in my mind, and in that moment, it became the answer to my prayer.

You will find a way. The road may not look the way you thought it would, but life is always guiding you along the path

Chapter Two

to your deepest fulfillment. When things don't go according to plan, don't be so attached to the destination that you forsake the signs and serendipities along the way. Be open to the guidance that surrounds you. Know that the obstacles are not really blocking you from moving forward, but are "detours in the right direction," as Gabby Bernstein says. Trust the path that unfolds before you. The soul's journey is not a linear pre-paved road to a clear-cut destiny. It is an ever-evolving spiral, weaving together all of your experiences, leading you to exactly what you need, at just the right time.

Converse with God

A few days later, I was back at work. Between flights, grooming staff come on board to clean the aircraft for the next trip. The cabin crew also walks through to see if anything is left behind for lost and found. Often we'd find a juicy *People* or *Vogue* magazine to keep us entertained for the next leg. Sometimes, we'd find a good book.

At the end of one particular flight, after surrendering my India plans and opening myself to guidance, I found a copy of *Conversations with God* by Neale Donald Walsch in a seat pocket. Intrigued by the title, I picked it up, brought it home, and read it cover to cover in one night. Written by an ordinary man who claims to converse with God, this book was revolutionary for me. What made the book so mind-blowing was that the author claims that we all have the ability to talk to God, if we still ourselves long enough to hear the answers and trust what arises.

Having grown up in the Roman Catholic Church, the idea that I could have a direct relationship with God without having to go through a priest or Jesus was refreshing. It's why I fell in love with yoga.

Wildfire Within

"When your choices conflict—when body, mind, and spirit are not acting as one—the process of creation works at all levels, producing mixed results. If, on the other hand, your being is in harmony, and your choices are unified, astonishing things can occur." Neale Donald Walsch

Unified, yoga, at one with Source. This is how I wanted to live my life. Body, mind, spirit all working together, moving as one. I had asked God/Goddess, the Divine Source for guidance and had always felt the presence of a Divine power in my life, but I thought I needed someone else to facilitate it. It couldn't be legit spirituality if it was happening outside of church walls or without prompting from a wise elderly teacher or guru, I thought. In my quest for meaning and purpose, I didn't always trust the insights that emerged following the deep questions of my heart.

I realized then that finding this book was part of receiving the guidance I had asked for. It was an answer to my prayers. It was God/Goddess's way of communicating with me that day. The guru I had sought to find in India, the one who would answer all my questions about the meaning of life and tell me my purpose, was apparently living closer to home than I had originally thought. The presence I was seeking was also seeking me and dwelling in my own heart.

The Flow of Grace

Newly single and looking to mend my broken heart, I looked for something else to do to fill the time I had carved out for India.

My budget was small and I wanted to find a direct flight to somewhere hot and exotic with yoga involved. After very little internet research, I found an inexpensive yoga retreat in Costa

Chapter Two

Rica, and impulsively signed up. I had no idea who was teaching or what to expect. The price was right and I was drawn to it. Something in my gut said, "This is it!" Three days later, I was on a flight to San Jose.

Landing in Juan Santamaría International Airport, I was approached by a small Costa Rican man with a sign bearing my name.

"Hola," he greeted me. "Your last name, Ayotte, is like the vehetable, Ajote," he laughed with his thick Spanish accent, walking me to his tourismo minivan. He was referring to winter squash. "Gustavo is my name. I will take you to your hotel in Jacó."

It was my first time in Latin America. I instantly felt at home, and bloomed like a flower in the warmth of the air and of the people. On the drive to Jaco Beach, Gustavo told me his life story, of how he was originally from Nicaragua and had moved to Costa Rica to have a more peaceful life.

"Too many problems where I come from," he said bluntly, shaking his head, recalling to himself all the bad things he'd left behind.

In that moment, I could relate to this small middle-aged Nicaraguan. We had something in common he and I: we were both running from pain back home, in search of solace somewhere else.

Gustavo dropped me off at the Poseidon Hotel two blocks from Jaco Beach, gave me his card, and told me to call him for a ride next time I came to Costa Rica. "You will be back, Chantal Ajote," he said smiling, as he drove away.

I checked into my room, and put my bags down as the sun was setting over the beach two blocks away. That night, the warmth of the breeze felt like a loving hug as I fell asleep to the sound of ocean waves crashing on the shore.

The retreat I had signed up for was not the typical luxurious yoga retreat. When I awoke and oriented myself the next morning, I discovered that the yoga classes would not take place at the hotel. In fact, none of the scheduled activities would happen there. A driver would pick up us, the retreat guests, and drive us to our daily yoga and surf lessons. In hindsight, I understand why I got such a price bargain on the retreat; it wasn't so much a "retreat" as a loosely pieced together yoga vacation. The man who organized and sold the package wasn't even a yogi. He was an old American expat, a washed-up hippy who was looking to make a quick buck. I figured this out after meeting him on my second day there, when he shared that, "Costa Rica is a sunny place for shady people."

Having now been in the yoga industry and run my own retreats for over ten years, I would never again sign up for this type of yoga retreat, knowing what I know about yoga and the importance of having skilled teachers. But at the time, I felt such a strong pull toward it and see now how it was me "finding my way," as the Indian Consul General had foreseen.

The other two retreat guests were a couple of girls from Upstate New York who had also bought this budget package online. We met at breakfast over *huevos rancheros* and *gallo pinto* (eggs, rice, and red beans), and bonded over the beauty of the land. Although not the most ideal setting as the hotel was located on a busy street surrounded by loud bars and partygoers, the hotel was decent, and I was happy to do anything that distracted me from the pain of my recent breakup. The hustle and bustle of the busy corner in front of the hotel provided enough entertainment, and I welcomed the sensory overload. Shortly after breakfast that first morning, a white shuttle van picked us up, and brought us to Vida Asana for our first yoga class.

Driving past Jaco Beach, we followed the windy cliffside road to the next beach town fifteen minutes away, Playa Hermosa. When we arrived at the yoga studio, we were greeted by

Chapter Two

Rosemary, an eccentric Argentinian mother of three who taught all the classes at the centre. It was her family's home, and they had recently built a small platform in the jungle where she could offer yoga classes to the locals, and to international retreat guests. Rose had wild curly blonde hair with streaks of grey. She was then in her late forties, with a wide lotus tattoo emerging from her cleavage. The sun-kissed deep lines on her face revealed that she had spent much of her life laughing in the sun. One of her eyes doesn't move as fast as the other when she turns her gaze. I later found out that she had lost her left eye surfing years before while living in Hawaii, and had a prosthetic in its place. Her joyous laughter pierced through any sadness I harboured; this was a woman who clearly had experienced intense trials in her life, yet was overflowing with a contagious exuberance for life.

"You have a beautiful practice, dahling; you are a teacher?" Rose asked enthusiastically after our first class in the yoga shala. I told her that I had done my first teacher training with David Swenson a few months prior, and would love to teach someday.

"You can come back here and teach any time," she proposed. "I need some help around here, so busy, always. I'm too busy with the children and their surfing and Alejandro ...."

I nervously laughed at the idea, flattered, and told her I would love to come back and teach for her someday.

We headed back to the hotel for lunch and our afternoon surf lesson with Miguel. That night, the phone rang in my tiny ground level hotel room. It was Rose. "Chantal darling," her deep Argentinian accent beckoned on the other end. "I have to go to San Jose tomorrow. Can you teach my class? There aren't a lot of teachers here and I know you will be a good teacher."

Surprised, but trusting her request, I seized the opportunity and agreed to help her out. I spent most of the night reviewing the primary series and memorizing the sequence I would teach in the morning to my two fellow retreaters.

The next morning, expecting that it would only be the three of us, we headed to the yoga shala for our daily yoga class. When we arrived, a dozen people were there for the class. It was my first time teaching a yoga class ever, and here I was on vacation, having to teach a group of fit and tanned surfer-yogis who, judging by their toned physiques, obviously knew what they were doing. Although I stumbled my way through the class and felt nervous the whole time, it was also exhilarating. I felt more alive than ever. Maybe it was the tropical breeze softly blowing through the giant palm leaves, or the adrenalin from my jittery nerves energizing me. Whatever it was, I knew that I had stumbled upon work that my soul longed to do on this earth—teach yoga.

Later that day, Rose called when she got back from San Jose and said everybody loved the class. She begged me to come back, to stay and eat and live with her family, in exchange for teaching classes. My heart jumped at the idea of living and teaching yoga in Costa Rica. I said yes, absolutely, and planned to return the following month.

The beauty of aviation life is the flexibility and freedom of travel that it offers. As a flight attendant, I could bid for my days off, and create my monthly schedules according to my preferences and plans that month. When I got back to Toronto after the yoga retreat, I began planning my work flying trips around my teaching trips to Costa Rica. I would bid to fly for two weeks in a row, and finish the month with two weeks off. Then I would bid the following month with the first two weeks off, and stack my flying for the last two weeks, and so on. That way, I was off for a month every other month. I would work like crazy for a month flying all over the world, then live and teach

Chapter Two

at Vida Asana in Costa Rica for the off months in between.

This went on for almost two years. Every time I went to Costa Rica, I would meet amazing teachers who were passing through—ashtangis on their way back from Mysore, yoga-celebrities from the US, and wise yoginis from South America. My time spent there was enriching and vivifying; an eclectic education on the many paths of yoga. I felt my soul come to life every time I set foot on the land of Costa Rica. It felt more like home than any other place I had dwelled.

During one of my early stays at Vida Asana, I was left in charge of the entire hotel while Rose and her family headed to San Jose for a few nights. I had spent enough time there that they trusted me with the operations of their family business while they were away.

"Don't forget to feed the dogs" she said, climbing into the passenger side of their old Volkswagen Westfalia a.k.a. the Surf Mobile.

"Oh, and Juan Carlos and his friend will be spending the night. He's like family and knows his way around. Put them in Villa 2," she yelled through the passenger window as they drove off down the long winding driveway, waving as they turned onto the road and out of sight.

The Earth Is Quaking

Of course his name is Juan Carlos, I thought to myself as I saw him step out of his truck a few hours later, surfboards tied to the back. Tall, dark and very handsome, he approached me smiling.

"Hola, hello," he said. "I am Juan Carlos, and this is my friend Eduardo. We are friends of Rose and Alex's." His gorgeous brown eyes fixed on mine; he looked pleased to meet me.

"Hola, I'm Chantal. I'm here looking after the place while

Wildfire Within

Rose and Alex are in San Jose. You guys can settle into Villa 2." I blushed, deeply attracted to him, feeling my body awaken to the visceral passionate heat he seemed to be exuding.

As he untied the surfboards from the top of his truck, he didn't hesitate to keep the conversation flowing, "Please, join us for dinner. We're going to an amazing restaurant in Jacó. It's the best. It would be a pleasure to have your company."

With my heart pounding, knowing I wouldn't be able to resist his charm, I accepted the invitation.

Heavy rain started to fall as we drove into town. The rainy season in Costa Rica is not like the rainy Canadian days I had known before. Rain drops the size of marbles splattered on the windshield as we drove down the highway. When we got to Jacó, we drove down a side street tucked away from the main tourist strip and went to a local spot that served the best seafood in town. Over ceviche and Imperial, Juan Carlos, Eduardo, and I laughed at how my last name was similar to the vegetable, and how the Spanish words for "lawyer" and "avocado" are also similar. Eduardo was a lawyer in San Jose, and Juan Carlos had just opened his own yoga studio. They had been friends since elementary school and were in town to surf for the weekend.

"So you like yoga?" Juan asked, deep brown eyes piercing into mine. We bonded over our love of the practice as the night went on, laughing and lingering on each other's every word. It was clear there was chemistry between us. Our connection was electric. Every cell in my body hummed to life in his presence. His sweet Spanish words melted the sadness of my recently broken heart and, like soothing dark chocolate, they filled the achy crevices with a delicious sweetness.

After dinner and a few mojitos, we picked up a bottle of wine and drove back to Vida Asana. Eduardo excused himself, claiming he wanted to get an early start on the morning surf, and headed back to Villa 2. Juan Carlos looked at me with a

Chapter Two

mischievous smile, wine bottle in hand, shrugging his shoulders and lifting his eyebrows, "Well, shall we enjoy this bottle together?"

I invited him into my villa, and led him outside my bedroom to the balcony overlooking the jungle, where we sat under the veranda watching the monsoon rains come down. Thunder rolled in the thick moist ocean air around us. Suddenly, the earth shook beneath us. We leaped into each other's arms and laughed at the intensity of nature's wild power. "Was that an earthquake?" I asked, having never experienced one before.

"Yes," he smiled. "And you know what earthquakes are?" he asked in all seriousness. "The earth having an orgasm," he whispered in my ear.

I laughed at myself falling for his seductive suggestions. But I could not resist. We held each other close and kissed in the thunderous rain. I felt every cell in my body come to life, awakened by the electricity in the air and the chemistry between us.

That first night together was magical. Lying in his arms, I felt like I had stumbled into a steamy Spanish romance novel and was suddenly the main character. I was twenty two and I had taken a Latin lover.

"You should come back, and come to my studio in San Jose. We have a teacher training next month. Come, as my guest. You can stay with me." He stroked my hair as I lay curled up in his strong arms, resting my face on his warm bronzed chest.

"Sounds amazing. I'd love to."

A few days later, I returned to Toronto a new woman. In love with where my life was going, India was the last thing on my mind. My recently broken heart had been restored by the balm of my new lover's embrace. For months, I travelled to Costa Rica on my days off, and studied with world-renowned teachers that passed through Juan's studio.

Wildfire Within

During my time there, I discovered and fell in love with Anusara Yoga, a style of hatha yoga created by an American yoga teacher. The word *anusara* means to "flow with Grace," or to "align oneself with the current of the Divine." The focus of the philosophy is to recognize that we are each embodiments of the Divine, and to joyously embody the sacred through our yoga practice and in our everyday life. Based on the tantric view that all of life is an embodiment of God, the goal is not to escape the suffering and the mundaneness, but to become deeply intimate with every moment, seeing it all as a manifestation of the One.

The first Anusara Yoga Teacher Training I did was with Kenny Graham and his partner at the time, Sianna Sherman. I had heard a lot about Sianna from Juan, and was told she was the top Anusara Yoga teacher to study with. She is lean and fiery, has a strong presence, yet a soft voice. She is both gentle and fierce, and I was captivated by her ability to weave mythology and philosophy into seamless stories that always stirred my curiosity to know more.

When I first met Sianna, she seemed distant and unapproachable, but suddenly, a connection emerged, which turned into a deep soul recognition for me, as though we had known each other before, in another lifetime. I felt a strong desire to learn more about yoga and continue my yogic studies with her. It felt like I had found the guru I had sought in India, except she did not come in the form that I expected (an old wise man with a beard) and she would never call herself a guru.

After the teacher training in San Jose ended, she invited me to the workshop she was teaching in Toronto a few months later. Unsure if I'd be able to attend, I said goodbye and flew back to Toronto the next day.

Three months later, the stars aligned again. I got the time off while Sianna was teaching in Toronto, and so I headed to her workshop at Kula Annex Yoga Studio. By now, it was clear to

Chapter Two

me that she was a deeply gifted and soulful teacher. Not only was she teaching yoga, but as a modern day priestess, she was masterfully weaving in ceremony, wisdom teachings of the Divine feminine, and prayer throughout all that she did. I felt a strong call to continue my studies with her, and completed my Anusara Teacher Training in San Francisco that year. Sianna became my main teacher, my mentor, my deep soul friend. I travelled to study with her and embraced every opportunity to learn from her.

Although I was never granted access to India in the way that I had wanted, Mother India gave me so much more, by opening up another way. Our life's path is not a straight and narrow road toward what we think we want or who we think we should be. The soul's journey moves in twists and turns, waves and spirals, forward and back, up and down; all for the purpose of deepening who we are. The blocks on the road are never really in our way, keeping us from the life we want. Rather, they are the way, the portals to our purpose, the gateways to our growth.

When the well-laid plans you make for your life begin to unravel, the disseminating moon is upon you. As her light begins to wane, darkness grows. The path before you becomes less clear, and from the outside, it may seem as though things are falling apart. Yet there is always a reason for the unravelling—the disseminating moon times are leading you back to your soul's purpose. When uncertainty of what lies ahead prevails, you must gather the strength from within you and fan the fire in your heart; it will light the way through times of growing darkness. Although we may feel lost at times, junctions of confusion force us to accept the mystery of life, and invite us to wander through this adventure in awe and with greater courage. You can never not be on your path. Every experience is for you to commune with; every step along the way is part of the unfolding of your destiny.

Wildfire Within

You will find a way. It may not look like what you had imagined, but you will always find a way. And in the end, it will be YOUR way, the only way you could ever take.

CHAPTER THREE

Embers: Learning to Let Go (Last Quarter Moon)

Last Quarter Moon: Listen within, turn inward, reevaluate, reorient toward letting go

"Each hell burns off more illusions. We go into the fire, die, and are reborn." Marion Woodman

Last Quarter Moon

As the moon journeys deeper into darkness, she moves through the Third Quarter Phase. Here, she must surrender to the coming winter, and turn toward letting go. The energy of the last quarter moon is one of reorienting ourselves toward the completion of a cycle, when only embers remain after the blaze, and the dissolution of what was is inevitable. As the outer form of what we have known continues to unravel, here we can turn our attention inward, and attune ourselves to the power of our intuition.

Chicago in the Autumn

At twenty-two, I thought I had life all figured out. I had found a way to immerse myself in yoga and do what I love. Flying to Costa Rica on my days off between international trips around the world, I was living my dream.

Enjoying the freedom of being untethered to a partner or children, I wasn't interested in finding the love of my life, let alone getting married. My plan for my twenties was to keep travelling the world, learning about yoga, and pursuing pure bliss.

Then I met Greg, and all my well-laid plans went up in flames, again.

After working a five-hour flight from Seattle to Toronto, I was scheduled to do a quick Chicago turn before a long stretch of days off, which I would spend teaching yoga in Costa Rica. Tired from the transcontinental flight I had just operated, I boarded the Embraer 190 E-jet with my fellow cabin crew, eager for the long day to end. I was assigned the R2 jump seat position, which meant that I would be working the first class cabin, and responsible for the pilots' meals and drinks.

Before passengers boarded, I prepared my galley, knowing I wouldn't have very much time to do so once in the air. As I smashed the ice bag onto the counter to break it up into smaller cubes, the pilots walked on. First on was the captain, who quickly said hello and ducked into the cockpit. Behind him was a young, tall, and very handsome dark-haired first officer. Taking his hat off, he tucked it under his arm, and extended his other hand to introduce himself.

"Hi, I'm Greg." My heart stopped and accelerated simultaneously. I had grown accustomed to working with older married men who were not my type and clearly off the market, so it was a delightful surprise to see such a young and handsome co-pilot for a change.

Chapter Three

"Oh hello, I'm Chantal. I'll be looking after you guys today. Let me know if there is anything you need," I answered, blushing as he smiled at me warmly.

"Same for you. Just let us know how we can make the flight enjoyable for you, and feel free to come up for a visit in-flight." He stepped into the cockpit, turning toward me with a smile before sitting in his right-hand seat.

As our eyes lingered on each other, I knew in an instant that the trajectory of my life had shifted. In that moment, I hoped the butterflies in my stomach would settle long enough for me to get through the flight without spilling wine on anyone's lap.

Flustered and nervously excited, I welcomed passengers as they boarded the plane.

It was common to visit the pilots in-flight during a lengthy voyage, but not something we flight attendants usually had time for on a flight shorter than two hours. But, as it turned out on that fateful day, we did not have a full passenger load, and there were only three people sitting in first class. After our initial climb to ten thousand feet and the seat belt sign went off, I served my passengers snacks and drinks, and finished what was usually a busy bar service in under ten minutes. I tidied up their empty glasses, hovered around them for a while, but nobody needed anything. In fact, two of them were sleeping, and the other was immersed in a movie. After putting everything away in the galley, I looked down at my watch and saw that we still had thirty minutes before beginning our descent into Chicago. Wanting to go say hello to Greg but not wanting to seem unoccupied, I stood by the flight deck door and hesitated before picking up the interphone to call up front.

"Oh, hi. Do you guys need anything? And, can I come up for a visit?" The captain unlocked the door, I entered the security code, and with coffees and salted almonds in hand, I let myself into my future.

Wildfire Within

The Embraer 190 E-jet is the smallest aircraft of the Air Canada fleet. I knelt down to squeeze myself into the very tight flight deck to chat. "So, how has your day been? Do you get to enjoy some days off after this?" the young dark-haired first officer asked.

"Well, actually yes. I'm going to Costa Rica tomorrow. I teach yoga at a surf retreat down there and spend most of my days off in Playa Hermosa."

"Oh, really? " Greg's interest piqued. He unbuckled the top two straps of his harness and turned toward me. "I love surfing. Maybe you can recommend some spots down there?"

"Sure, I'll give you my email and I can send you some links to the best surf spots in Central America." I wrote my email down on a small piece of paper fed through the data link printer, the little machine that sends messages from ground control. As we chatted, eyes locked into each other, air traffic control called from Chicago. Clearly distracted, the young first officer kept missing calls from the tower. The captain rolled his eyes and said, "Don't worry, Greg. I got this." As we started our descent into Chicago, I remembered that I had to secure the cabin for landing, and headed back to my galley, my heart fluttering from the flirtatious encounter.

The flight home from Chicago to Toronto was a full one. When we landed and all of the passengers disembarked, I was happy to see that the co-pilot was still there. We walked the long walk through Pearson International Airport to customs together, talking the whole time about our love of travel and the ocean. Then he offered me a ride home and I accepted.

When we arrived, he pulled up alongside my Bloor Street flat, a three-bedroom apartment I now shared with two other flight attendants. "Well, thanks for the ride. Maybe I'll see you out in the surf some time."

"Definitely" he responded.

Chapter Three

As I opened the door to my apartment, he drove away. Unsure about if and when we would next see each other, I was hoping our paths would somehow cross again.

The next day, I flew to Costa Rica, and thought of Greg the whole time. Things with Juan Carlos quickly fizzled out, as they usually do when they begin so passionately. We were no longer lovers, but we remained good friends.

Greg did send me an email a few weeks after we'd first met. This began our friendship, which eventually became romantic a few months later. Our relationship began somewhat long-distance, as he was transferred to Vancouver whereas I was sharing my time between Toronto and Costa Rica. As our budding relationship blossomed, my trips to Central America slowed down and I began spending all of my days off with him. Eventually, we found ourselves in the same city long enough for him to propose; it was only eight months after we started dating. We married a year later, on September 12, 2009.

Rooting Down

After the wedding, Greg and I moved into a Toronto condo that was built directly above the High Park subway station. During the first few months of wedded bliss, I took a six-month leave of absence from Air Canada in order to pursue teaching yoga full time. Every morning, I rode my bike down Bloor Street to the Kula Yoga Annex, and enjoyed the creativity and consistency that teaching regular classes provided.

Once that leave ended, I was granted another three months off, and it was then that we decided to relocate to the West Coast of Canada. We were both granted base transfers, and moved to Vancouver to live near the ocean, which I had always dreamed of doing, and to be closer to family. We were offered a long-term house-sitting opportunity in White Rock, an ocean-side suburb an hour outside Vancouver, and I began teaching yoga in the city.

When my second leave of absence ended, I had to make the difficult decision of quitting yoga teaching or quitting flying. I wanted to do both, but I wanted to master the craft of teaching yoga more, which I knew in my heart was not a part-time pursuit. Flying was still fun, for now, but Greg and I knew that we eventually wanted to start a family, and would not both want to be flying when that time came. If I quit teaching to go back to work as a flight attendant, I would have to release all my classes and later start over, having to rebuild what I had already begun creating. In my heart, I knew I wanted to commit myself wholly to teaching.

It was one of the hardest decisions in my life. Faced with two different paths before me, I had to choose just one, the next step of my journey. I feared regretting the decision to leave a stable job with benefits, but the thought of denying my dreams was even more frightening. I knew that resigning from Air Canada would mean becoming more dependent on Greg, financially and otherwise, and that made me nervous. I didn't like the idea of relying on someone else to pay the bills.

The fear inside me told me to hold onto the job, in case the relationship or the yoga career didn't work out. The benefits were good; I had a pension; it could be my back up, I told myself. But the more I looked at why I wanted to hold onto the job at Air Canada, the more I realized that fear was running the show. As Marianne Williamson says, "We can either make a decision out of fear, or out of love." Knowing that I wanted to live my life from a place of love and expansion, rather than one rooted in fear and contraction, with Greg's support, I handed in my resignation letter to Air Canada. At the ripe age of twenty-six, I retired from flying. That was in June 2010.

Suddenly, my whole scheduled opened up, and I was free to

Chapter Three

study and teach yoga as much as I wanted. But instead of feeling liberated, I felt a knot in my stomach, an energetic hangover from the bold life-changing move I had just made. An internal tension emerged when I realized what a gypsy soul I was. Now, unable to travel for work, I had to get used to having two feet on the ground, all the time. As though my wings had been clipped, I felt a heaviness come over me that I would pretend was not there.

In the sobering weeks of uncertainty after I left my stable and adventurous career behind, I questioned if the heart was really something to be trusted. Swept up in new love and dreams of becoming a global yoga teacher, I was now faced with the task of actually making those things happen. I soon learned that teaching yoga full time is not as easy and simple as I had imagined. There's a lot of hustle, hard work, and competition involved, running around the city teaching twenty classes per week, all in an attempt to get my foot in the door in more studios, to get enough people to come to my classes so I can get good time slots and a decent schedule, and hopefully, earn enough money to pay the bills if I am lucky. Being a yoga teacher in Vancouver was like being an actress in Hollywood auditioning for classes in an oversaturated market and trying to catch a break.

The hustle was real, but so was the grace that continued to guide me day by day. I did enjoy teaching yoga, and I chose to focus on all the opportunities that were opening up before me, rather than on all the tense uncertainty that comes with being self-employed.

When I'd question whether I had made the right decision to leave the comfort of the corporate world, I would remember the wise words of India's General Consul: "You will find a way." I always trusted that somehow, everything would work out, that Life, God, and the Universe knew the longings deep in my heart that wouldn't lead me astray. I believed that my dreams of teaching yoga and travelling the world would provide a road map to living the life I longed for. Although I feared the future and had a pang of regret in my gut after leaving the airline, it felt as though, no matter what I chose, there was no "wrong way." I could only choose from many amazing paths, each with twists and turns, challenges and triumphs. I had to trust that whatever path my heart was urging me to follow was the right one for me.

Becoming a Householder

I come from a long line of amazing French Catholic women who got married young, and had lots of babies. My grandmother had nine children — NINE! At age forty-five, she unexpectedly became a widow when my grandfather died in a train accident. With no income of her own and no driver's license, my Mémé had to find a way to make it work. She learned how to drive and got a job at an insurance company to provide for herself and feed her family. No matter how dire things got, as a devotee of Mother Mary, she was a woman of faith, and always believed that Love is the most powerful force in the Universe. Through the way she lived her life, my grandmother taught me about resilience, strength, faith, courage, and unconditional love.

As the youngest of those nine children, my own mother experienced how hard life was without my grandfather around. As a child of the sixties, Mom was encouraged to find herself a good man to provide for her, and that's exactly what she did. My mom met my dad in high school, was married at nineteen, and had three kids by the time she was in her mid-twenties. So, as a young girl, I thought that this is just what women did. Subconsciously I grew up thinking that the purpose of my life was to grow up, find the love of my life, and start a family.

Chapter Three

When I started flying and travelling the world at nineteen years of age, I realized that there was more to life than having children. As my passion for travel increased, my desire to find a husband lessened. In fact, marrying was the last thing on my mind. The freedom I experienced in my early twenties made me question if I ever wanted children at all. I thought that perhaps one day, later in life, after I had seen all the places I wanted to see and done all the things I wanted to do, then maybe, I'd be ready to settle down.

Naturally, that's not the way life played out. When I met Greg, I knew that if the day came when I would want to get married, I'd want it to be with him. Deeply in love and seduced by the promise of "happily ever after," I said yes when he proposed.

But at twenty-five years old, I was not ready to be married. Neither was he. No one ever is, we were assured; being married is how you learn about marriage. So we took the dive and, soon after, realized why the pastor who married us compared the wedding day to the first day of kindergarten, not graduation day. It was only the beginning of learning what it means to truly love one another, not the culmination of our love.

We got married the traditional way in a Christian church. Greg had rediscovered his Christian faith while flying in the Arctic, and it had since become an important part of his life. He wanted to get married in a church, and to wait until we were married before living together. He was somewhat countercultural with his desire to do things the traditional way, which was one of the things I loved about him. He wasn't like the other guys I had known. He was sincere, he had integrity, and I trusted him deeply. We moved in together after we were married, and that's when we began to understand what our pastor was talking about. The wedding day was only the beginning, and being married was a lot harder than anyone had ever warned us.

We knew we had different worldviews and that our dreams

did not always align. I wanted to travel the world, live abroad, and become fluent in Spanish. He wanted to buy a house, pay off our mortgage quickly, and begin saving for retirement. I wanted to live in an urban neighbourhood where we could walk everywhere and not depend on a car to get around. He wanted to live outside the city, somewhere quiet near the ocean, where he could windsurf on his days off. I believed the earth is sentient, the Universe is always conspiring in our favour, and that our vibration attracts our reality. He believed in a Father God who sent his only son to save us.

In the beginning, our differences made the other interesting. We did not see our diverse opinions about the nature of life as major chasms in our partnership. I was a yogi and I sought union in all things—especially in my marriage. In an effort to be selfless and create harmony, I often translated dogmatic rules about how to be a good Christian, or things we'd hear preached at church, into mystical meaningful teachings. Many times I silenced my resistance to Greg's literal interpretation of biblical verses, fearing that my voice would spark another argument about what the original authors of the scriptures really intended with their allegories. We had many common interests, but our spiritual orientation was not one of them. Both intrigued by the unseen powers that be, many loving dialogues turned into ignited debates about the nature of God. It didn't take long before we started avoiding the subject all together—the evangelical Christian and the tantric yogini lived side by side with no resolution in sight.

On the Sundays Greg was home, we'd attend church together, going through the motions, making small talk with the other newly married Christian couples we'd met in suburbia. From the outside, we were the picture-perfect couple. On the inside, I felt my soul was dying. I knew in my heart I did not belong there. Although it was the lineage of my upbringing, Christianity did

Chapter Three

not feel like home. But as a yogini, I always sought to bridge the gap, to find the commonality, and to look for the good. I was a tantrika, and the challenges of my relationship were part of my path as a householder. I viewed all of our difficulties as grist for the mill of my spiritual development, and I sought to transcend our troubles. As skillful as I was at pretending our differences did not matter, the fissure in our beliefs was becoming more of an insurmountable crevasse in the bedrock of our relationship.

Follow the Dream

Two years after meeting Sianna and only three months after resigning from my stable corporate job, I awoke from a vivid dream in which I was her apprentice and assistant. In the dream, I saw myself working alongside her, learning all the wisdom ways, and teaching many people, feeling confident and overjoyed to be immersed in yoga. When I woke up, I felt so energized, happy, and revitalized. The dream had been so clear and felt so real that I felt more awake and alive in the dream world than I did on waking. It took me a few minutes to reorient myself to my reality. Still enraptured by the vivid clarity of the dream, I immediately wrote Sianna an email to say hello and tell her about what I had just experienced.

Not expecting a prompt response, I was delighted when she wrote back twenty minutes later. It turned out, her former assistant had just resigned, and she was looking for a new one to take his place. Sianna was not at all surprised by my message. She admitted to being very active in the dream world and had asked Spirit to call in the right person. After a joyful easy chat, she asked for my resume. We set up an interview, and a few weeks later, I became her tour manager and apprentice. The trajectory of my life changed once more.

By literally following my dream, a new possibility emerged. I was given the opportunity to combine my passions, and I began travelling globally with a world-renowned teacher to study the art of yoga and assist at festivals and conferences all over North America. I attended retreats in Bali and Italy, and apprenticed at trainings in Paris and San Francisco. I brushed shoulders with the world's most renowned yoga teachers, some of whom later become my dear friends. The years that followed became the most enriching and formative yoga training I could have ever imagined.

It is during those in between times—after one thing has ended and the next has not yet begun—that we must have the most courage. In nature, during the fallow times when it appears as though nothing is happening, new seeds are being incubated, rebirth is stirring below the surface. Although the in-between or liminal spaces are full of uncertainty, they are also full of possibility. If we can muster the courage to let go gracefully, we can free and open ourselves up for something new to emerge.

The Householder's Path

Through my studies of Anusara Yoga with Sianna, I was introduced to Tantra, not the "sexualized" new age version we have come to know in the West, but the deeply feminine path of intimacy with life, a full embrace of the journey.

Tantra refers to a set of teachings, practices, and tools for both spiritual liberation and deep fulfillment in worldly daily life. Through the tantric lens, all of life is a manifestation of Divine energy. Our bodies, our problems, our tissues, and our issues are not obstacles to our liberation, but doorways to our innate freedom. Nothing is rejected on this path as "not spiritual." Everything is a portal to God. The point of Tantra is to become more embodied, more fully awake as humans. Like a knowledgeable sommelier who tastes the subtle nuances of

Chapter Three

the soil the year the grapes were harvested, *tantrikas* (those who practice tantra) attune to the sacred notes underlying every experience, and seek to taste all the *rasas*, the flavours of life. As scholar Douglas Brooks, PhD, puts it, "life is a gift to be savored, not a problem to be solved."

Often described as the householder's path, the essence of tantra reveals that God is not an external patriarchal force living out there in some distant plane removed from creation, judging our every move. Spirit is not separate from matter, but deeply infused into every atom in the Universe. God/Goddess is not a powerful force outside ourself, but the very ground we walk upon. The air we breathe, the body we inhabit, the medium of our existence, and awareness itself are holy. God/Goddess can be felt within every breath and known in each moment. There is nowhere that Divine consciousness is not.

"All sentient beings are simply different forms of one divine consciousness, which looks out at a universe that is its own body. All things are part of one, vast energy field, vibrating at an incalculable number of different frequencies. All that exists, has ever existed, or will ever exist, is one infinite divine being, free & blissful, whose body is the universe, whose soul is consciousness. You are not separate from God/dess and never have been. Indeed, you are the very means by which she knows herself." Hareesh Wallis

Through the tantric worldview, embodiment as a human is not seen as a hindrance to spiritual liberation, but rather the celebratory expression of Divine union. Creator's nature is to create, and she continues to create through us. We are not separate from the sacred heartbeat of life, but are in holy relationship with the power that pulses through everything. We are embodiments of the force we call God, and are co-participants with source in the ever-unfolding story of creation.

In tantra, the feminine principle is sacred, and revered as the source from which all life flows, the Great Mother. Masculine and feminine, heaven and earth, solar and lunar, spirit and matter are necessary polarities that co-exist in balance to form the whole. Nature, creativity, and diversity are celebrated as the full expression of Divine Love.

The word *tantra* itself means "to weave." It also means "to stretch" and "to expand across a threshold." The imagery often used to describe its elegant philosophy is that of a loom. Imagine hundreds of diverse threads, woven together to form a beautiful tapestry. They stretch from one side of the wheel to the other, individually expanding to create a unified whole. The tapestry is symbolic of our own life, woven of the diverse richness of every experience. Through warp and weft, joys and sorrows, our soul expands. By stretching ourself into being, we grow into our full expression.

The word *tantra* also means "to protect." The root "tan" means to stretch, and "tra" is to protect. And so it is said that tantra stretches and spreads wisdom that saves. Tantra is so called because it stretches our awareness and expands our capacity for joy. In our essence, we are holy, whole, and healthy; our true nature is Divine. But we are also forgetful beings who suffer from cosmic amnesia, it seems. The teachings and practices of tantra serve to remind us of who we are. Like drinking water or waking from sleep, remembering who we are is not something we can do once in our life and be done with it. It is a daily task to embody presence and see the divinity in all things.

Tantric Sadhana (spiritual practice) is not about reaching a perfected future state, but rather is about dissolving whatever blocks your heart from experiencing the perfection of each moment. As Shambhavi Sarasvati says in her book *Pilgrims to*

Chapter Three

Openness, "Tantra does not urge us to skip over the being human part. The only way out is through, and the way through is full of beauty." Tantra is all about empowerment. Ultimately everything on our path can be used as a catalyst for becoming who we're meant to be in the world. Everything is happening for us, not to us. No matter how gorgeous or how painful, it is all gift.

Remembering My Own Light

Shortly after Greg and I got married, we moved to the West Coast, I left the airline, and I began working with Sianna Sherman, my yoga teacher and mentor. My work with Sianna was invigorating and enriching. Through it, I was always meeting new people and learning empowering wisdom teachings. Some of my duties included managing her global tour, scheduling her events, booking international travel, and negotiating contracts with yoga studios around the world. I was often on the road travelling with her and assisting at workshops, festivals, and conferences internationally. On weekends I'd chant mantras and learn about tantric goddesses who slay demons. At home between touring, I'd struggle to connect with my husband, arguing what Jesus meant by "I and the Father are one." The contrast between my domesticated life as Christian wife and my adventurous, free-spirited goddess-filled work life became stark. I began feeling as though I was living two lives: one where I could be who I really am, and one where I had a loving partner and all the material comforts, but did not feel like myself. It felt as though I had squeezed myself into a tight corset—it was once fashionable and may have looked really good, but it was stiflingly uncomfortable. I couldn't breathe.

As time went on, Greg and I continued to support each other's work, but began living somewhat parallel lives, side by side but not really involved in each other's worlds. I continued my attempts to understand and truly believe Christian theology, in an effort to connect with my husband spiritually.

Early one spring, a work trip took me to Costa Rica to assist at a yoga centre in Nosara. Sianna was teaching with another yoga teacher, Amy Ippoliti, and with Douglas Brooks, a Srividya Tantric scholar who would be leading afternoon lectures on Tantra. Over a hundred people travelled to attend this gathering on the Pacific coast, where the wild jungle of the tropics meet the serene white sandy beaches of the Nicoya Peninsula. The sunsets in Nosara are pure magic. Watching the gorgeous golden glow illuminate the sky with shades of pink and yellow hues as it disappears over the horizon is spiritually illuminating. Just as the sun sets every day, so too will our light eventually fade. The journey west that the sun takes toward darkness is a beautiful reminder of our own soul's trajectory.

One of the many people who journeyed to be on this yoga retreat was Juan Carlos. It was the first time we had seen each other in five years, since we had last been lovers. Now a married woman, I had to ignore and suppress the scintillating chemistry that still ran between us. His flirtatious gaze and sensual touches were met with an awkward frigidity, a forceful distance I had to create between us for fear of what I would feel if I didn't keep my energetic guard up.

Seeing Juan Carlos was a welcome reminder of the person I had been. We had spent enough time together and knew each other well enough to talk about how we were feeling, and how much our lives had changed. We laughed at how unnatural it felt not to embrace the other while in each other's presence, but he respected that I was committed to someone else.

Although I remained faithful to my husband, and nothing happened between Juan and me during the retreat, it was the first time I saw within myself the potential to stray, and the first time I recognized all the ways I was contorting myself to

Chapter Three

fit into my relationship. It scared me to think that I would be capable of betraying my husband. Yet what frightened me more was realizing how much I had betrayed myself, since marrying Greg. Running into Juan Carlos reminded me of the person I had been not that much earlier: passionate, wildly curious, and on fire for life. I was a fun-loving free spirit, enraptured with the Great Mystery. In an effort to be a good Christian wife, I had severed and unconsciously shut down parts of myself that are essential to who I am. Only two years into becoming a wife, I was no longer being myself within my marriage. From fear of judgment because of being misunderstood, my soul had dimmed her light in order to fit into her new surroundings. Only embers of who I knew myself to be remained.

After the retreat ended, I returned home with a resolve to channel into my marriage this renewed sense of passion within myself. I went home to Greg, determined to really be myself again and to spice up our life together. I loved him deeply and wanted our relationship to thrive, and I realized that it would be up to me to create the conditions for that to happen. So when I got home, I embodied the sexy passionate self I had rediscovered during my time in Costa Rica. In the first few weeks back home, a breath of fresh air revitalized our relationship. We reconnected, and it felt as though we were growing closer together emotionally and spiritually.

Then, as things always do when you least expect it, life took another major turn.

From Tadasana to Savasana

Shortly after coming home from Costa Rica, I spent a week assisting Sianna at a teacher training in San Francisco. We finished the seven-day teaching intensive with a weekend workshop taught by Sianna and Darren Rhodes, where we did all the poses in the Anusara Yoga syllabus, from beginning to end.

Symbolically, Tadasana or "mountain pose" is done at the beginning of practice. It is standing in full, embodied presence, with both feet grounded, crown lifting toward the sky, heart open and centred as the mid-point, the meeting place of heaven and earth. Savasana or "corpse pose" or "death pose" is the last pose at the end of a practice, symbolic of death or the end of a cycle. Yogis practice Savasana at the end of every class, as a means to practise conscious letting go; something we must all learn to do, if we are to live a good life. From Tadasana to Savasana, every class represents an entire life cycle. From emergence into the world, our birth is practised at the beginning through child's pose. Then we move into the early active years of young adolescence, marked by active warm-ups done early in class, followed by maturing into adulthood with the stability of standing poses, flowing into claiming our throne as an elder when we take seated poses, and finally, practising our own death with corpse pose when we practise dissolving back into the source of life.

Every yoga class can be practised symbolically as the embodiment of this great cycle that is mirrored throughout all of creation, including the turning of seasons, the blooming of flowers, and the phases of the moon.

During that weekend workshop, on Friday we completed Anusara Yoga syllabus one, which took almost six hours. On Saturday, we were in session for eight hours practising more intermediate poses, and on Sunday we spent five hours exploring the most advanced yoga poses, which most of us could not get into without the help of a friend.

I flew home after the workshop feeling very tired—my body had never done so much yoga and I had never before pushed myself into poses the way I did that weekend. Also glowing for

Chapter Three

another reason, I was eager to get home to take the pregnancy test I had bought at Walgreens on my way to the airport. My period was over two weeks late. Unsure if it was due to all the travel or to the yoga I had been doing, I was anxious to go home and find out.

When I got back to our apartment, I quickly greeted Greg with a kiss and darted into the washroom to pee on a stick. Surprised by my hasty entry, he walked into the bathroom to see if I was okay. Shocked by his unannounced intrusion, we looked at each other quickly, then he scanned the bathroom floor and saw the box and instructions to the pregnancy test scattered on the ground. His whole face lit up. "Are you pregnant?" he asked, enthused by the prospect.

"Well, we'll soon find out," I said, waving the pee stick in the air to dry, in hopes of getting the results faster. Two minutes later, the results were in. With a little digital word appearing on the mini screen, our whole Universe shifted: PREGNANT.

Greg and I looked at each other and smiled with disbelief. We ran into each other's arms elated, laughing, and sharing tears of joy. After some time, the initial shock and excitement wore off, and my tears of overwhelming joy turned into sorrow. I blamed it on the hormones, but deep down, I was grieving the upcoming loss of my newly ignited freedom. I knew I wanted to be a mother someday, but not yet; I was just beginning to reach a level of recognition in my career that I thought was necessary to become the internationally renowned yoga teacher I dreamed of being. Things with my husband were somewhat rocky; we lived comfortably alongside each other but lacked true emotional or spiritual intimacy. The thought of becoming a mother was a sobering reality check that would mean some big changes in my life. Most of all, I wouldn't be able to travel any more, and I'd become somewhat cut off from the global yoga community I had started to feel so at home in. And even more importantly, Greg and I would have to make things work if we wanted to raise this child together.

The Tomb Is the Womb

There is a saying in the Celtic priestess tradition: The tomb is the womb, and the womb is the tomb. Something must die for something new to be born. Birth and death cannot exist without each other. When a woman becomes a mother, part of her life is over. She is no longer a maiden, carefree and untethered by worldly responsibility. There is a natural grieving that must happen when we go through times of transition, to fully step into the next phase of our soul's evolution. We must consciously release an outdated way of being, so we can be ready for what's emerging through us, what is yet to come.

When I became pregnant, I wanted to become the best mother I could be, yet I still wanted to hold onto a part of my life that allowed me the freedom to do as I pleased. I was not ready to submit all my dreams to the transformation that was beckoning me forward.

As my due date drew near, Sianna and some of my girlfriends in San Francisco created a beautiful blessing way for me. A blessing way is a traditional Navajo ceremony designed to honour a woman's passage into motherhood. Different from our modern day baby showers that focus on the arrival of the baby by showering the mother with gifts and supplies she'll need once baby has arrived, blessing ways are intended to mark the woman's initiation into motherhood, offering her prayers and blessings for a safe and healthy birth. It's a beautiful way of marking the transition from maiden to mother, and helps the mama to step into this next phase of her life more empowered and spiritually prepared. My own blessing way was in Sianna's living room in the Marina District in San Francisco. Surrounded

Chapter Three

by gorgeous *murtis*, deity statues Sianna had collected over a lifetime of world travels, my soul sisters showered me with blessings, songs, and prayers for a safe passage into motherhood. We ate delicious chocolate and fruit, and they sang over my belly as they massaged my hands and feet with healing anointing oils. It was one of the most nourishing experiences of my entire life. That evening, I felt so blessed to be a woman. Honoured to be the carrier of life, a vessel for new possibility, I felt like a goddess amongst goddesses, and knew the Divinely feminine power within me.

After my blessing way, I realized that becoming a mother is a transformational threshold, an initiation that I would get to walk through. What a privilege to be brought into the circle of motherhood, I thought. I knew that I would be changed through it, but I had no way of knowing how transfiguring it would actually be. I anticipated the birth with great excitement, and could not wait to experience bringing a human into the world.

It was during the labour that the lump was discovered. My old self died the day I became a mother. My womb became the tomb to whom I had been. And it was in that dying, in entering that tomb, that I also entered the womb, the fertile darkness of the Great Mother. I would be reborn into who I am meant to be.

Surrender

Receiving a cancer diagnosis is a traumatic event marked by shock, disbelief, and fear. In the wake of such a life-changing event, one is left paralyzed by the weight of uncertainty that follows receiving such devastating news. Like a wildfire blazing through our perfectly planned life, difficult times force us to surrender to the wisdom of the flames. Life as we have known it is destroyed, and all we can do is let it happen.

Wildfire Within

In nature, a wildfire sweeps through the forest, consuming everything in its path with a blazing intensity that cannot be suppressed. Leaving a trail of destruction and ash, the forest floor is no longer recognizable; it is not what it used to be. When I found out I had cancer in my body, it felt like an intrusive fire devouring me from the inside. There was no escaping or taking flight from my body. There was nowhere I could run to where the wildfire was not. If you try to suppress a wildfire, it will rebel with bursting flames that reach higher and wider, leaping from one tree to the next, as though it knows deep inside that there is a purpose to its transformational hunger. When I found myself consumed by the fire, I couldn't bypass the heat; I had to let it burn.

Finding the lump during labour catapulted me into the tumultuous world of cancer. Suddenly, between changing dirty diapers and cuddling my son, my days were filled with oncology appointments, x-rays, and daily visits to British Columbia's Cancer Agency. Everything changed so quickly; from one day to the next, I no longer recognized my life or myself. Some days I'd feel so scared and angry, I'd want to curl into the fetal position and close my eyes, hoping to wake from the nightmare I was living. But I couldn't allow myself to indulge in self-pity. I had a newborn baby to care for, and a life to save—my own. Suddenly, the world had become a dark place. A deep gloom swept over me, the sky seemed forever grey; my heart became heavy, filled with grief and the despair that comes from being so disoriented, no longer recognizing who I was. I yearned for the life I had known before, for my joie de vivre, which had vanished with the realization that I might die before I had the chance to really live.

In the yoga tradition, Kali is the dark goddess of death and destruction. She wears a necklace made of the skulls of all the demons she has slayed, and she licks up the blood from the

Chapter Three

severed heads. The heads represent our egoic mind, and the demons she slays are all the voices inside that hold us back, that keep us from living into our full potential. Kali Ma is fierce and often feared, but ultimately she represents the necessary death of transformation. She is the loving force that dissolves the fixed forms we cling to, so that we can create something greater. Purified and freed from all the falsities we have about who we are, when we experience times of darkness, we are being cooked in the fire of her love. She sees our fullest potential and will not allow us to stay small in a world that needs us to shine. When Kali cleans house, it's always for our highest good.

Just as Kali is both calamitous and life-giving, a wildfire appears to be a force of pure destruction and devastation, but it is a natural, necessary and, in essence, deeply nourishing part of nature's health and sustenance. The ecological benefits of wildland fires often outweigh their seemingly negative effects.

Wildfires burn away that which is invasive, diseased, and toxic. By removing undergrowth, more sunlight reaches the forest floor, which supports the growth of native species. Fire liberates nutrients locked within old plants, creating nourishing ash, which is released back into the soil for new life to emerge. New buds burst forth from the charred earth with deeper roots, brighter shoots, and a resolve to grow. Expansion happens naturally, when we understand that death and destruction always precede creation. Simply put, a wildfire allows more light to pour in and through the living matrix that it transforms.

Like embers fading back into earth after the fire, I surrendered to the process of recalibration. In choosing to let go of the person I had been, and of the resistance I was holding toward my own life, I harnessed the liberating power of the last quarter moon. By turning my attention inward and attuning to

Wildfire Within

the soul voice inside, I reclaimed the nourishing dark part of the lunar cycle. In so doing, I would come to remember my own cyclic nature and trust that this dissolution was part of my evolution.

CHAPTER FOUR

Ashes: Dying to be Free (Balsamic Moon)

Balsamic Moon: Let go, trust fate, meditate, sacred memories, wisdom, ebb, descent

"The world is as you see it. If you do not like what you see, change your prescription of glasses." Baba Muktananda

The Balsamic Moon

Before returning to complete darkness, a subtle sliver of the moon's light glows as the balsamic moon. Named from the root word of "balm" or "salve," the balsamic moon—the final lunar phase before the new moon—is about assimilating wisdom to soothe the soul. Her invitation here is to reflect upon and absorb all the lessons gathered from the recent blaze, before stepping into rebirth.

Fire has long been seen as the element of transformation. Not only does it burn away that which we no longer need, but it also brings nourishment to that which is yet to come. After a fire has extinguished itself, the remaining ash holds within it nutrients for new life. A year after a wildfire takes place, a resilient species of gourmet wild mushrooms called "morels" grows from the ash. Morels, prized by gourmet cooks and considered a delicacy among foodies, literally rise from the ashes the springtime after a forest has been ravaged by fire. Mushroom hunters travel from all over the world to harvest these wildly robust fungi. Due to the nutrient-rich ash that fuels their potential, morels flourish after a fire.

I didn't yet know what possible benefits could come from the devastation of my cancer wildfire, but one thing was clear. I could play the victim, see it as the worst thing that ever happened to me, and be devoured by the flames. Or, I could walk through the fire as an empowered yogini, be alchemized by the process, and use the heat of the crisis for my own liberation.

Our view, the way we look at life, shapes and colours our experience. Our perspective can limit or liberate us; it can deplete or fortify us. The way we choose to look at things will ultimately determine how our life unfolds.

Not long after I found out I had cancer, I allowed myself to wallow in despair for a few days. Playing the victim seemed like the most obvious response when life handed me a lemon. I was a new mother, only twenty-eight years old, living my dreams, and madly in love with life. Now, it was all being taken away from me—I'd have to undergo cancer treatments and lose all my hair. I might not live to be thirty or to see my son grow up. My dreams of living a long healthy life were shattered, and there was nothing I could do to change my situation. I continued to imagine the worst-case scenario and feel sorry for myself, pitying the tragic turn of events my life had taken.

I soon realized that, if I was going to make it out alive, this approach was not going to work. Seeing myself as the helpless victim was not going to get me through this, or help me get well; quite the opposite, it only made me feel worse, more exhausted, and more sick.

Chapter Four

When the severity of my situation hit, I realized that no one would save me from this mess; no one could heal my body for me. I was the only one who could affect change in my wellbeing. I knew that if I want to live long enough to see my son grow up and maybe even long enough to one day meet my grandchildren, I would need a different approach. I couldn't control what was happening around me, but I could consciously choose how to view this chaos, and be deliberate about how I would walk through it. As the old cliché goes, I would try to squeeze any possible goodness out of this tragedy, and be nourished by the process.

As a yogi, I had spent a decade practising different poses designed for different purposes. Some poses help open your hips; others strengthen your shoulders. There are *asanas* ("yoga poses") that increase lymphatic circulation and others that elongate your spine. Many poses are named after animals, warriors, sages, and elements found in nature. One of the benefits of practising a wide variety of yoga poses, in addition to toning the whole body, is that it allows you to see life from many different vantage points. How does it feel to root down like a tree or move like a snake? Each pose has its own unique vantage point through which to experience the world. Every posture is essentially a different perspective through which to view life. More than just a static position to force your body into, each pose is an invitation to be intentional about the way you inhabit your body and your life; about what posture and position you take in your world. *Merriam Webster's* dictionary defines posture as "a particular way of dealing with or considering something; an approach or attitude." Practising yoga then becomes about choosing your attitude, your stance, and the way you live your life.

I couldn't change the fact that I had cancer, but I could still choose my posture. When I practise yoga, I try to feel the energy power inherent in all of the beings I am embodying: the rebirth of the snake, the courage of the warrior, the wisdom of the sage. Practising warrior pose in the devastating midst of chemo treatments awakened within me the remembrance that I am on a sacred journey. At different points along the journey, different qualities were required, and the years I had spent on my mat had helped me access all the ways of being I would need to rise to the challenge. No matter what the outer pose looked like, I decided to see myself as the heroine of my own life. The chaos of cancer was happening *for* me, not *to* me. Through the fire, I would be fortified, and become my own fortress.

The Heart of Recognition

As soon as I made the decision to see the cancer as happening for my greatest good, I began to ask the Universe to show me what I needed to do in order to heal. I knew that this health crisis was a spiritual crisis. It wasn't so much about changing the foods I was eating (I am a vegetarian) or tweaking my exercise regime (I do a lot of yoga). This was an initiation, a trial by fire to transform me on the deepest level.

Instead of fighting against life, I started asking it for help. No longer convinced that I was living in an abundant Universe that had only my wellbeing in mind, I was forced to surrender my naïve notion that we alone control our reality. How could this popular theory be true, I wondered. Did I do this to myself? Why would I create my own cancer? What was this really about? If life was trying to teach me something, what was it?

Up until then, in theory, I had believed that life was made of sacred energy. The yogic teachings that I love so deeply espoused an expansive Universe that vibrates, that pulsates and hums with the heartbeat of love. I understood that tantra is ultimately about stretching ourself into new possibilities,

Chapter Four

and integrating the light and the dark. Learning about these philosophies was beautiful and energizing, and somewhat easy. Living tantra is a whole other matter. It is easy to believe that life is a gift and everything is happening for me when things are going my way. Of course, I could feel and see the Divine in moments of laughter and the setting Costa Rican sun. But how, I wondered, could cancer be as holy as my joy? How could my hardships and heartbreak be manifestations of Divine energy?

Driven by my quest to discover a deeper purpose to my pain, I fell to my knees and cried out to whatever Source Energy was out there, begging to be shown the way out of the darkness I was feeling. There was no going back to the way things used to be. Life was pulling me forward, to a place I did not want to go. There was no getting around it, the only way out was through.

When news of my cancer diagnosis reached my wider circle of friends in the yoga community, people reached out from all over the world, offering any support I might need. It's hard to know what you'll need as a new mom who is beginning cancer treatments. People sent me scarves, flowers, sympathy cards, and inspirational poems. I was even given breast milk, because when I'd start chemotherapy treatments, I would no longer be able to breastfeed my baby. Women that I didn't even know would pump extra milk and send it in frozen bags to our apartment. Looking back now, I see how we can draw nourishment from many places. We joked that Ben had many mothers. The Great Mother comes in many forms.

Most of the time, I would just cry when receiving these gifts, still in shock and disbelief that it was all really happening. Waves of anger and helplessness would consume me, and I'd collapse in tears on the bathroom floor of our small Yaletown apartment, totally at a loss for how my life had fallen apart so quickly. What did I do to attract this? Why me? Why now? My mind would sink into despair, spiralling down a deep paralyzing vortex of victimhood.

But one gift sent early on by my first tantric philosophy teacher, Hareesh, awakened me to see my fate in a new way. When he first got news of my diagnosis, he was teaching at a friend's yoga studio in Toronto. We arranged a call after his lecture, and when he called from Kula Yoga with the owners of the studio beside him, I immediately asked them all how they were doing, attempting to take any attention off my situation. Clearly they were calling to console me, but I did not want to appear like a weak or faulty yogi who had somehow failed or done my practices wrong and ended up with cancer.

It was then that Hareesh noticed how much I was putting other people ahead of myself. By addressing everyone else on the call first, without giving them space or time to acknowledge the reason for our conversation, I was putting others' wellbeing before my own. It was an insignificant detail that might seem benign at first, but that revealed a deeper belief I had about myself.

"It may sound harsh, but always putting others' needs before your own is a form of self-hatred. Not placing as much value on your needs as you do on others', is not giving the Divine spark within you as much importance as you give the ones around you," Hareesh noticed. His words took me by surprise, but they resonated. Could it be that, deep inside, I did not really value myself?

He then gifted me his online course on an ancient tantric text called the *Pratyabhijna-hrdayam* (in English, "The Heart of Recognition"). Desperate for some deeper wisdom to cling to, I gratefully accepted and began listening to the teachings at night when my husband and son were asleep. Instead of reading books about cancer or scouring the internet for answers, I turned to

Chapter Four

an ancient Indian text written in the ninth century, and found meaning in the madness I was living.

Beyond the pseudo new-age affirmation that "all is well," the recognition that the text speaks of is ultimately about seeing oneself again, as we really are. It describes how we are all made of Source energy, but in the stepping-down process from blissful-loving consciousness to human form, we have forgotten who we are: a contracted form of vibrant luminous fullness. The whole world is made of blessing energy, and all that happens is conducive to our growth and success. Tantric practice is ultimately about seeing the Divine in the midst of chaos, and the chaos itself, which is sometimes necessary, as a reminder to us of that truth.

Listening to these teachings on my way to chemotherapy treatments reminded me that there was another way to walk through this tragedy. Perhaps there was more going on than I could perceive with my limited view of what life is supposed to be like.

What if, as all the tantric teachings alluded, even this, a cancer diagnosis, were somehow a blessing? Could the darkness that had come over me also be a gift? Although I wasn't yet clear on how the dissolution of my perfect life could possibly be for my greatest good, I was curious what my teacher Hareesh meant when he said, "This is as God as it gets." Could I learn to release the resistance, dissolve the tensions from my body and heart, and be open to the possibility that this too was Divine? That it was happening for me? That there was a deeper purpose to my pain, and I could still feel the scintillating magic of life, even while going through cancer treatments? All of these questioned swirled in my mind, but I was also filled with fear. I couldn't help but feel that yoga had let me down, had not fortified my body against this inner invader. Could I trust anything I had ever believed, about how our actions matter? And if so, could I really affect matter, my body, the world around me, through my thoughts, my desires, my prayers?

Again, I had been really good at being happy and spiritual, and believing all the yogic teachings when life was going my way. Now, I had to learn what to do with the ugliness of fear and rage, the physical and psychological pain of poison being pumped into my veins, and life not going the way I had planned.

Before our phone call ended, Hareesh recommended that I read *Dying to Be Me* by Anita Moorjani. The story is the author's experience of dying of stage four Hodgkin's Lymphoma (the same disease I had), having a near-death experience, then returning to her body, which became cancer free a week after she had entered the hospital.

At first I was resistant to reading about a woman who had died from the same disease I had. But I was curious about what her experience had taught her, in hopes that I could apply it to my own condition, and maybe even heal myself through it. As I read her story, I recognized a common thread we both shared. She too had been exposed to many diverse and sometimes conflicting belief systems (Christianity and Hinduism), and had allowed her fear of letting other people down guide her daily choices.

In her book, Anita describes her experience of "the other realm," of how we are all made of love and that, ultimately, life is to be enjoyed. There is nothing to fear, she says. "Each of us is an integral part of the greater unfolding tapestry that's continually working toward healing the planet. Our only obligation is to always be true to ourselves and allow."

Immersing myself in ancient and modern stories of remembering our true nature, I felt myself being guided back to health. Day by day, I learned to accept the life I was living and released my need for it to look a certain way.

Chapter Four

This Is Happening for You

As I leaned into accepting my new reality, I released the resistance, and stopped pushing against what was. Instead of trying to control the conditions of my growth, I decided to allow the unfolding of my life and search for the blessings in my situation. One by one, day by day, they continued to reveal themselves.

On a visit to my naturopath's office, I met a vivacious woman who would continue to shape my course. Sitting beside each other in big upholstered chairs receiving our weekly doses of vitamin C intravenously, we exchanged small talk and shared why we were both there. "I've been told I have colon cancer, stage 3," she said, " but I know exactly what it's about and I know it will be clear in less than six months. I know I have some forgiveness and letting go to do."

Surprised by her self-confidence and optimism about her condition, I asked her curiously, "What do you mean? How do you know for sure?"

I longed to have such clarity about my own circumstances. "My medical intuitive confirmed what I knew I needed to do, to clear this blockage in my body," she responded.

"Medical intuitive?" I asked. "What is that?"

She went on to explain that a medical intuitive is someone who understands the emotional or energetic root cause of an illness. She gave me the name of her intuitive and, as the nurse took the IV out of her arm, she went on to explain that she is an MD who has her own medical practice on Granville Street in Vancouver. "Be sure to contact her," she said, leaving the room. "We won't be seeing each other here again, because soon enough, this will all be behind us" The fortuitous lady smiled, with a reassuring wink as she left the room. Recognizing this as an answer to my prayer for guidance, I contacted the medical intuitive as soon as I got home.

When I met Dr. Divi Chandna a few weeks later, her big

brown eyes and loving smile were already more uplifting than the sombre oncologists I had become accustomed to seeing. She explained that in addition to being a medical doctor, she listens to the body's intuition and gives voice to what my body already knows deep inside my bones. I immediately relaxed and trusted her completely. Not only is she a qualified MD, but she is East Indian and loves yoga. She embodies ancient wisdom and personal power, and understands the importance of the body-mind-spirit connection. Dr. Divi spoke my language, bridging the worlds of medicine and spirit.

After an in-depth physical and subtle body assessment, Dr. Divi described the energetic qualities of the last few years of my life. "Your spirit was soaring," she explained, "then something happened, two or three years ago, and you shut down. Your immune system and sense of self shut down with you."

I explained to her, as she knew nothing of my past and my personal life, that I married around that time and that I have struggled to be myself completely in my marriage. I shared with her how conflicted I was about trying to fit into the religious box I had married into. I loved my husband deeply but saw all the ways he was bound to an outdated view of religion and, in trying to save our relationship, I had lost myself, shrinking my worldview into one that was not my own.

"There is much truth and beauty at the heart of Christianity," she continued, "but it is not your path. Rather than trying to change yourself or your spirituality to look exactly like your husband's, see yourselves as two wheels on a wagon. You're both separate, but connected; different entities but moving in the same direction. Chantal, this is happening for you to be who you really are."

Her words struck a chord and echoed inside me. "This is happening for you to be who you really are." In that moment, I understood what my body was asking of me. It wasn't

Chapter Four

looking for the perfect diet or the right supplement. My body had turned against itself, just as I had turned against myself. In trying to be someone I was not, I was killing the light within me that longed to shine. Of course I was experiencing dis-ease. I was un-easy in my own skin, forcing myself to fit into a mould of who I thought the world wanted me to be — the flawless Christian wife and perpetually blissful yogi, with everything figured out, always perfect and happy. My body was not the enemy; it was my greatest ally, alerting me to the madness I had been living in pretending to be anyone other than myself.

So who was I, if not the wife, mother, yogi, cancer patient I had become? Who was I dying to be? Dr. Divi's words were like a key that unlocked a newfound desire to live. Of course I wanted to make it through this ordeal and see my son grow up. But even more than that, I wanted to know and liberate the one inside me that was dying to be free.

La Vie En Soul

With a new resolve to discover who I really am, beyond all the identities I had created, I started to view all of the things happening around me as manifestations of a Loving Energy that had only my highest good in mind. I was here to be me, and so I needed to discover who that me is. I had been cooked in the fire, not to be destroyed, but to be strengthened, the same way a potter places earth in the kiln to become fortified earthenware. The heat is the transformative element that turns clay into ceramic, so it may become a strong vessel, adding not only function but beauty to the world.

For years as a flight attendant, I had been used to viewing the world from above. From high in the sky, cities and problems below disappear as your vantage point broadens. Leaving a rainy city, I always liked that point in flight when the airplane breaks through the clouds into clear blue skies. A perennial reminder that the sun is always shining; we just don't always see it from where we are standing. Now unable to get on a plane and jet-set across the world, I had to connect to a different kind of sunshine, an inner fire that burned within my own being.

One of my favourite songs has always been Edith Piaf's "La Vie en Rose." In it she describes seeing the world through rose-coloured glasses, through the eyes of love, and the sweet elation that comes from being held in the arms of a beloved. What if I could see "La Vie en Rose" not just as a classic love song reserved for romance? Could I adopt this way of seeing life, and learn to fall in love with my constraining conditions, my cancer, myself? Instead of viewing life from above, beyond the here and now, ascended past the pain and beauty of the present, could I see the transmuting flame of love from within the fire? Could this cancer be a loving crucible for my soul's calcination?

As I began to view my situation from a deeper place, I tried to infuse it with the spirit of "La Vie en Rose." My new mantra became "seeing la Vie en Soul," looking at life through the eyes of my innermost self. I needed to accept and even fall in love with life, exactly as it was—imperfections, sleepless nights, rocky marriage, cancer, and all. I had to learn to embrace and embody who I really am, before I could really heal.

Becoming Soul Fluent

"Seeing la Vie en Soul" meant I had to reorient my relationship with life and view everything as uniquely designed for my soul's evolution. Like any new relationship, I needed to get to know my soul again and to remember how to communicate with this most essential part of myself. I had

Chapter Four

to learn and remember the language my soul speaks, if I was to nourish her and help her bloom.

One of my favourite cities in the world is Paris. The gorgeous architecture, the aesthetic elegance in the streets, and the romantic feeling in the air always awaken within me a joie de vivre, and the feeling of deep appreciation for the beauty of life. I have always felt at home in Paris, as though I belong there, or have lived there in another life. Growing up, we spoke French at home. Speaking my mother tongue always feels more familiar to me. I love the way Parisian French words roll off the tongue and the romantic flavours they leave in the mouth. Something inside me wakes up when I speak French; I feel more vibrant, more alive, more like myself.

Like speaking another language, we must learn to understand and translate the way our soul speaks to us, if we are to embrace ourselves on the deepest level. Sometimes when we invoke a higher power and ask for guidance on our path, we expect miracles in the form of angels descending from heaven or the thundering voice of God to articulate the answers we seek. But the revelations we are searching for are not revealed in English or French or in any dialect we can hear with our ears. The soul speaks not in words. She lets herself be known through feeling, symbols, beauty, and a visceral knowing in our bones. Dreams, imagery, and imagination are the vehicles for the deep wisdom we call on, so it's important that we open ourselves to all the ways we are being guided throughout our life, and pay attention to the signs.

Living through a cancer diagnosis is a journey weighted with fear. Walking to the cancer agency on my way to chemotherapy one day, I noticed how much fear I was harbouring after learning that I would also need radiation treatment. If I don't do it, will

Wildfire Within

the cancer come back? If I do it, will I develop a secondary cancer later in life? Am I doomed either way? Fear, fear, fear, fear, fear .... My mind was consumed with thoughts of the worst possible outcome and all I wanted was a guarantee that once this was over and done with, I would be happy and healthy for the rest of my life.

Then, something beautiful happened—as I was crossing the Cambie Street Bridge by foot with my arms crossed over my chest, a white feather floated down from the sky. As though moving in slow motion, it descended gently flowing right in front my eyes. Taken by the simple beauty of the feather, I stopped in my tracks and watched it float to the ground. I picked it up, and looked up toward the sky in search of a bird or flock from which it fell. The sky was clear blue, not a bird in sight. To most, this would seem meaningless and insignificant. But in that moment, time stopped, and intuitively I knew it was a sign, a love note from Spirit. As though fallen from an angel's wing, that feather reminded me that on the deepest level of my being, I was already healed, loved, and taken care of. In that moment, I knew it was a sign from the Universe, reminding me that even through my pain, I was being supported by an unseen higher source that was always there, and trying to make itself visible. All I had to do was open my eyes and see the way it was speaking to me. The sign itself was not that remarkable. It was but a moment of peace, a sigh of relief, a subtle shift in perception. It was also an answer to my prayer for guidance. In that small parenthesis in time and space, I felt the vastness and Love of Spirit.

From then on, I began seeing feathers everywhere, in the most unusual places. I noticed them at doorway thresholds, tucked in people's hats, and in my drawers. Soon after, I learned that in many ancient traditions feathers symbolize healing, freedom from fear, great vision, and transformation. When I began to

Chapter Four

view la vie en soul, feathers became my symbol, one of the ways Spirit was speaking to my soul, lovingly leading me on.

That fateful day, when I got to the cancer agency, I had a renewed sense of courage and deep trust in the goodness of life. I greeted my dear friend Laurie, who had come to sit with me through my treatment, and she was taken aback by how lighthearted I was. I told her about finding my sign, and that I knew everything was going to work out for my greatest good. We laughed as we walked into the cancer agency, calling it the "spa" and acting as if we were just two girlfriends going for a healing infusion treatment, spending an afternoon together, and reconnecting over coffee. And that's exactly what it became.

As I sat through my chemotherapy treatment, I felt a rush of love for life. I changed my perspective and started to see all the ways I was being shown love. I felt it through my friend and her caring words, through the nurse who tenderly administered the healing medication, through the warm golden sun peeking through the clouds.

When you open to see all the ways love shows itself throughout the day, you begin to see it in every experience, even the ones that aren't so comfortable. Somehow, in the midst of my darkness, I was always given just enough strength to endure, just enough energy to do what was needed. On the days that I struggled the most, when I didn't think I could go on, I'd see a feather, and somehow, strength would find me.

Just as the balsamic moon gracefully surrenders to the dark, I wanted to let go of my fear, trust fate, and embrace the wisdom that arose when I dared descend into the wild unknown. Moment by moment, day by day, my path to healing was revealed. Take a deep breath, go for a walk, laugh, pray, cry, listen, and feel with my heart. There was no prescription to follow. I had to feel my way out of the woods. I let my intuition be my guide, and slowly I remembered the language of my soul.

Wildfire Within

When I listened deeply, my soul did not speak to me in revelations or money-back guarantees. The answers to my deep questions were not downloaded in an instant. Instead, she spoke to me in sweet feelings of relief, glimpses of joy, and the soothing sensation of hope that comes over a person when they remember that this too shall pass.

I was tired of clinging to the limiting conditions of what I thought a beautiful and happy life was supposed to look like. Clearly trying to force my way to freedom was not working for me. My fixed agenda was futile. I didn't know how it would all end, if I would recognize myself or my life, or whether I was still going to be married when it was all over. All I knew was that the tapestry of my life was not complete. There was a thread I was carrying, a purpose to my presence, a soul gift that was an integral part of the whole. I didn't yet comprehend the sacredness of the web I was weaving. But I knew that I wanted to live to find out.

Chapter Four

Even in the Struggle
by *Tara Sophia Mohr*

Even in the struggle, you are loved.
You are being loved not in spite of the hardship, but through it.
The thing you see as wrenching, intolerable, life's attack on you,
is an expression of love.

There is the part of us that fears and protects and defends and expects,
and has a story of the way it's supposed to turn out.
That part clenches in fear, feels abandoned and cursed.

There is another part, resting at the door of the well within, that understands:
this is how I am being graced, called, refined, by fire.

The secret is, it's all love.
It's all doorways to truth.
It's all opportunity to merge with what is.

Most of us don't step through the doorframe.
We stay on the known side.
We fight the door, we fight the frame, we scream and hang on.

On the other side, you are one with the earth, like the mountain.
You hum with life, like the moss.
On the other side, you are more beautiful:
wholeness in your bones, wisdom in your gaze,
the sage-self and the surrendered heart alive.

Source: *The Real Life*, poems by Tara Sophia Mohr
www.taramohr.com/poetry-book/

CHAPTER FIVE

Rebirth: Embrace the Dark (New Moon)

The New Moon: Plant, intuit, open, truth, dream, surrender, release

"The greatest sin is to dry up." Hildegard of Bingen

"Pain is the breaking of the shell that encloses your understanding." Rumi

"The cure for anything is salt water: Sweat, tears or the sea." Isak Dinesen

New Moon

Everything begins in the dark. In her darkest phase when her light is no longer visible, the moon's power is in her most hidden form. Like the fertile darkness of soil, she cloaks her light to regenerate herself, and prepares to birth herself once more.

In the Celtic earth-based traditions, the darkest part of the year is celebrated as the new year, or the beginning of the cycle (between Samhain and Winter Solstice) because they recognize that everything begins in the dark. From the seed in the dark soil to the fetus in the womb, all new life emerges from the dark. Times of darkness are not feared but welcomed, for when we find ourselves here, we know that the dark contains the seed for the light. It holds the full potential for anything to emerge.

Snake Medicine

In nature, we can witness the power of rebirthing by looking to the sacred snake. Throughout ancient cultures, snakes were revered as symbols of femininity and fertility, for just like the womb, the snake sheds her skin and is reborn again and again. Snakes naturally move close to the earth, and sensuously feel their way through life by attuning to the rhythms and vibrations they hear with their whole body. In yoga, the snake represents Kundalini Shakti, the creative power within each of us that is said to reside at the base of the spine. Yogic practices are designed to cleanse the physical and subtle bodies so we can awaken to our innate creative energy—our inner snake power, our ability to recreate ourselves. Shamanic and priestess traditions have long honoured the serpent, even though it was eventually demonized by the church, for the deep archetypal feminine power of rebirth she embodies. Like the new moon, the snake, and wild nature, the Divine Feminine is always regenerating herself. To know the sacred feminine is to remember the power of rebirth. Death always gives way to new life.

Dark Days of the Soul

A few months after my angelic feather encounter on the bridge, I found myself on the other side of chemotherapy treatments.

Near the end of my six-month regime, I was feeling progressively more tired. The treatments are cumulative and their effects are felt more intensely as the chemicals accumulate in the body. The first few months of treatments were relatively easy. I still had stamina, a positive outlook, and all my hair. Weekly vitamin C infusions and a daily meditation practice kept my energy levels and mood up. But as the third month dawned, my body started to weaken, and the luminous life force within me began to dim. When I started waking up to chunks of fallen hair on my pillow, I decided it was time to shave my head.

In solidarity, Greg shaved his head too. In fact, it became a family affair. Every week we would shave each other's head in the bathtub, with Ben in his baby chair looking on. We laughed at how all three of us were sporting the same bald baby look and wondered if he would ever remember these bizarre early days of his life. Dismayed at how quickly things had unraveled since Greg and I first met, back when life was fun and carefree, it was a daily effort for me to see the good in our situation. No longer free to jet-set the globe together (he was still flying but I was earthbound by a baby and weekly appointments), we struggled to connect as sleep-deprived new parents going through cancer treatments.

Greg coped with the fear of losing his wife and the mother of his new child by taking on more work. Providing for his family was the only thing he felt he could control and do for us during this difficult time. After all, we still had to pay the rent and buy groceries; somebody still needed to bring home the tofu bacon. When he wasn't flying, he was in the home office on his laptop, head down, buried in volunteer union projects he had taken on as a way of keeping himself sane.

Men in our culture are not taught how to deal with emotions, let alone with difficult ones. Instead of acknowledging or expressing how they feel, they are told to stay strong and soldier on. As the shaky ground of our relationship became even more vulnerable under the weight of new parenthood and the stress of a life-threatening illness, Greg built walls of work around himself.

Chapter Five

Although he was becoming increasingly occupied with his work, he was also evolving into an amazing father. When we found out I wouldn't be able to breastfeed, Greg bought a deep freeze to store all the extra bags of breast milk I was pumping early on plus all the breast milk we would receive. We called the milk acquisition and storage operation "Greg's Dairy." At night, he woke up to bottle-feed the baby so I could sleep away the nausea and deep fatigue that consumed my bones. We did what we had to do, to get through the turmoil we found ourselves in; his way was to numb the discomfort of fear by staying very busy, to check things off the to-do list, and to turn away from feeling his emotions at all.

Married only two years, we had a new baby to care for, and a health crisis to deal with. We did not have the life experience or tools yet to face this with any kind of forethought or grace. Catapulted into the disorienting cancer-land circus, we flung ourselves into survival mode, and forsook all of the wonderment and joy that new parents normally experience. Our time together was not spent revelling in each other's company or planning for the future. We no longer talked about trips we dreamed of taking or conversed about matters of the heart. All of our energy was funneled into doing only what was needed to get through each day. Stifled by the suffocating weight of daily medical appointments, dirty diapers, sleepless nights, and a bleak prognosis, the intimate connection and romantic flame between us all but extinguished itself.

When faced with fear and especially when our survival is at stake, our sympathetic nervous system takes over. The body reacts to threat by initiating the fight, flight, or freeze response. We each have our own way of dealing with different stressors in life. He flew away, literally and emotionally; I fought to stay alive, and our tender relationship froze under the chill of what we were facing.

The Girl with the Feather Tattoo

When chemotherapy treatments ended, radiation was scheduled to begin, a daily dose for eighteen days straight. Finding out I needed radiation crushed me. With chemo at least, I knew the chemicals would move through and out of my system eventually. But radiation felt like an irreversible attack on the centre of my being. It felt as though I was going to be branded on a cellular level, because the radiation was literally going to be targeted toward my heart and chest area.

The week before radiation began, I mustered enough energy to go to my friend Meghan Currie's yoga class. When I walked into her full class, she welcomed me with a big loving hug, which is when I noticed the tip of a feather tattooed over her shoulder.

"My daily feather!" I exclaimed, laughing to myself at how my feather would show up in the most peculiar places.

"Isn't it amazing?" she asked, turning around so I could see the rest of the large design, which wrapped all the way down the back of her arm.

I told Meghan about how feathers were my symbol from Spirit, and that I was thinking of getting a tattoo of one as well.

"I know a guy—we'll come over tonight!"

Anyone who has ever met Meghan knows what a radical free spirit she is. Unconventional in every way, she is one of the most creative and courageous people I know. She makes her own clothes and her own music, and teaches the most wildly invigorating yoga classes. Inspired by her boldness, I spontaneously agreed to let her arrange the whole thing.

After her intense class, most of which I spent in child's pose, I headed home and looked at images of feathers that I liked. I pulled out a gift that another friend, Trisha Wilson, had sent the week earlier from Nelson, BC; it was a gorgeous eagle feather

Chapter Five

she had found on the beach. She sent it to me wrapped in a dark woven-cotton cloth, with a love note explaining that she had seen it and immediately thought of me, and wished for me the strength and great visionary power that the eagle medicine represents. Unbeknownst to her, I already had my thing for feathers. That's another way they would come into my life—by mail!

That night, after I put Ben down to sleep, Meghan came over with her friend Jamie, the tattoo artist she had met at a party the week before. As Greg was out of town for work, they came to our apartment so that I wouldn't have to arrange for a sitter.

I welcomed them in and we sat for a while, looking at images of feathers that I liked, then talked about where I wanted to put it.

"Well, I'd really like it on my forearm … but that seems quite bold," I hesitated, worried of what my mother-in-law or husband would think. "I was also thinking it would look nice on my foot," I tilted my head to the side and looked down at my pointed foot, envisioning what it would look like there. "What do you guys think?" I looked up and asked Meghan and Jamie.

"I feel like the foot is safe, as in, not many people will see it, and you'll be able to hide it. The foot is definitely the safer choice … it's safe … if that's what you're going for," Meghan responded, with a mischievous twinkle in her eye that invoked my inner wild woman.

"Safe" was a feeling I had outgrown many months earlier. Any illusion of certainty or control had been shattered for me, when I heard the words, "You have cancer." Playing safe was too small for what my soul needed. It no longer fit. Like a cage restricting my ability to fly, in living my life by always trying to please other people, I had clipped my own wings. I was no longer willing to box myself into an inauthentic way of being, afraid of what others might think, perpetually trying to keep everyone around me safe and comfortable. Now, I was willing to ruffle a few feathers by tattooing one onto my body. It was to serve as a reclamation of my liberation, a daily reminder that my soul is free, and that Spirit is always present and guiding me. And so, I chose to put the feather tattoo on my forearm.

We lit a candle and smudged my living room with sage. Within minutes, our little twenty-third-floor Yaletown apartment became a healing sanctuary. Getting my tattoo was a sacred ceremony, a threshold crossing, a reclamation of my unique radiance. It was my own way of awakening the warrioress within—the one within me who does not fear what people might think, but instead chooses to love and live life on her own terms, unafraid of being her most authentic self.

Elated and empowered by the experience, I also wondered what Greg might think of my new ink when he came home the next day. Having been raised a good, wholesome, clean-cut suburban Christian boy, he didn't have any tattoos and was not particularly fond of them.

After coming home and dropping his luggage off, he accompanied me to my radiation preparation appointment. As we sat in the radiologist's office waiting for the doctor to arrive, we chatted over what he had done the night before, during his layover in San Francisco. "It was a bit of a late night at the duelling piano bar" he shared, smirking and explaining that he and his captain had stayed until the end of the show to see which of the two pianists would be applauded as the winner.

"Sounds like fun," I said, pausing to think of how I'd recount my own recent late night out. "Well ... I had a bit of a crazy night too."

Surprised that I had done anything of interest beyond feeding the baby, changing diapers, and sleeping off the blues, Greg looked at me intrigued. I rolled up my sleeve and revealed my big bold new feather tattoo. A shocked look washed over his

Chapter Five

tired face. He took my arm to examine it more closely, then looked up and said, "Wow, Chant, it's beautiful," with heartfelt sincerity.

Taken aback by his positive response, I felt a rush of love for my husband in that moment, a feeling I had forgotten since we had found ourselves in this cataclysmic mess.

Moments later, the doctor arrived. She explained that after looking at my CT scans, the radiologists would position my body on a table and mark the areas targeted for the radiation treatments that were scheduled to begin the following week.

"How do they mark my body?" I asked.

She hesitated a moment. "Well, it's important that the radiation is targeted to the correct and very specific part of the body every time. The only way to ensure that is by marking reference points ... permanently." She paused, in fear of upsetting me with what she was about to say. "We tattoo them on."

Having just gotten my feather tattoo the night before, I laughed at the perfect timing of it all. Instead of fighting the process, I giggled to myself, feeling a newfound sense of courage. "That's fine," I responded smiling. "I like tattoos."

Surrender Some More

The week I got all my new tattoos (four in total!), I felt myself really surrender, for the first time on a visceral level. Contrary to the defeatist connotation that word might invoke, "to surrender" is not about becoming passive. It is not a lazy response or merely giving up when things get tough. Quite the opposite, surrendering is an active response to life. It is deliberately choosing to channel your life force in the most optimal way. Like opening a tight fist after it has been clenched, surrendering is about loosening your grip so that you can be present to life's guidance and the wisdom of your intuition, moment by moment.

When I surrendered to being a cancer patient, a willingness to face my own death arose, and pent up energy that had been used to fight against my condition was suddenly liberated, free to move and flow toward my healing, rather than just being consumed by my suffering. I wanted to evolve and grow from it all, and listen deeply to the voice of my soul. Rather than impose my own agenda about what I thought my life was "supposed" to look like, I opened myself up to the Creative Power of the Universe.

Mantra Medicine

A few weeks after radiation started, renowned tantric scholar Paul Muller-Ortega, PhD, was passing through Vancouver, offering a meditation workshop, and *diksha*, an initiation for committed meditators.

I had wanted to study with Paul ever since hearing Sianna rave about his elegant articulation and practical dissemination of ancient tantric teachings. Meditation was a practice I was becoming more accustomed to and was learning to appreciate, ever since becoming a cancer patient. Since treatments began, my body had become more tense and rigid. The natural flexibility I had always taken for granted had been replaced with achy bones and shortness of breath. Although I wasn't doing as much physical yoga in the way of asana practice (yoga poses), every morning I sat for ten minutes of meditation as a way of reconnecting with the one within me who is whole and luminous, untouched by disease and decay. On some days, she was hard to feel, but if I sat long enough, I could feel her steady presence below the dark and stormy waters of my mind.

The ancient tantric texts suggest that a seeker on the path

Chapter Five

cannot progress along her spiritual journey without receiving *diksha* through receiving an activated mantra from her teacher. The idea behind this ancient ritual is that the benefits of all the practice, hard work, and insights of our teachers can be given to us through mantra. Like a multivitamin packed with nourishing nutrients, a mantra is a sound vibration infused with grace and love. When we recite a mantra, quietly, internally, or out loud, the energetic qualities of the vibration reorganize our nervous system, sending new messages to our cells.

In the tantric tradition, teachers or gurus of old would initiate their disciples by giving them a personal mantra to work with, dependent on what the aspirant needed to grow. These mantras are "charged," as it were, with the grace of the guru, and they serve as catalysts for clearing away negative thought patterns, and awakening the Shakti or spiritual creative energy within. Students would spend a lifetime learning from only one spiritual teacher, and the potent wisdom pearls of their teacher would be condensed energetically and downloaded into *sutras* (short potent teachings) and mantras, passed down orally over hundreds of years. Mantras are not just ancient, meaningless sounds that you recite. They affect consciousness, and consciousness affects matter. Mantras move energy and are liberating vibrations, keys that unlock the creative potential within us.

Although I was feeling an aversion to gurus and I was already going through my own initiation, I was drawn to the more subtle and powerful practices of yoga. Since viewing my encounter with cancer as a soul initiation, I longed for ceremonies and rituals that outwardly symbolized the inner transformation I was going through, to mark the threshold I was crossing.

When Professor Paul Muller-Ortega came to town, I seized the opportunity to receive my very own grace-activated mantra. He told us stories of the early days he had spent at the ashram in India of his guru, Maharaji. Excitement and frenzy always ensued at the ashram and crowds gathered whenever the four singers from Liverpool came to study with Maharaji in the late sixties. Professor Ortega was one of his senior students at the time and one of the main teachers to bring Transcendental Meditation (TM) back to the West. He was part of the TM community for decades before he took all that he had learned from his guru and evolved his own particular style of meditation he called "Neelakantha Meditation." In this particular style of meditation, the mantra given to you by your guru is meant for you and you alone. Activated mantras are uniquely calibrated for your own growth. Because they are personalized seed sounds of potential, their potency grows over time as they are repeated inwardly in the fertile ground of your mind and heart. They are not meant for everyone, nor are they beneficial to others. As tillers of the soil before becoming planters of a seed, students must commit to their practice and be strong enough containers to really reap the benefits of working with an activated mantra.

Traditionally when you receive an initiated mantra, it is said that what keeps your mantra powerful is keeping it sacredly to yourself. It is not meant to be shared or spoken out loud. Like a personal internal vow, an activated mantra is meant for you alone. Although being initiated with a personalized sacred sound is a potent practice, it is only one of the many healing and liberating ways of working with mantra. There are many mantras that can be used freely without the guidance of a teacher. These mantras will support your journey to the heart of who you are. Don't wait for a guru to free you. Initiate and liberate yourself.

That particular meditation immersion with Professor Ortega was five-days long. In the morning, I would sit, study, and sing with my *kula* ("spiritual community") at Inner Space yoga studio in Gastown. After lunch, I'd go to the BC Cancer Agency for radiation. I walked into the radiation ward feeling powerful

Chapter Five

and protected—strengthened by the mantra I had been given. When I would lie on the table to receive radiation, I chanted *"Om Namah Shivaya"* and visualized a healing light beaming into my chest, zapping all the cells that were no longer needed. I thanked my body for the intelligence to know the difference, and bathed my living cells with love and gratitude for healing and regenerating themselves with so much ease and resilience.

When I really began working with my mantra on a daily basis, I started noticing how much chatter was going on in my mind, when I wasn't being deliberate about my thinking. During that time, so much of it was fearful or judgmental chit-chat. If I wasn't internally repeating my mantra to myself, what was my default state? How was I talking to myself and what was I thinking about most of the time? We don't think of our inner dialogue as mantra, but the thoughts we think to ourselves affect the way our cells behave. If we are always critiquing ourselves or fearing a certain outcome, our brain is sending anxious signals to our body, drowning our cells in stress hormones.

Mantras affect matter, both the matter of our cells and in turn the life we create around us. Just like the food we eat has an effect on our health, the words we repeat inwardly and outwardly shape the worlds we inhabit. We may not consider the thoughts we think of as mantras, but our inner dialogue—what we say to ourself—becomes the soundtrack of our life. Like a beautiful musical instrument, our physical body emits the music of our soul. If the strings are out of tune and our mind is discordant with negative thinking, it will be harder for the sweet song of our essential self to flow. The thoughts we think, the words we speak, the way we inhabit our body can either inhibit or enhance the radiance within us. Mantras become medicine when they serve to tune our soul strings and clear the blocks that keep us from remembering who we really are.

Twice Born

In yoga, there is a pose called *Svarga Dvijasana*. Often translated as "bird of paradise pose," the literal meaning from Sanskrit is "twice born." All birds are born twice: once as an egg and then a second time when the bird emerges from its shell. In order for the bird to really live, it must break through the safe little shell in which it first dwells. A scary and painful process, perhaps, and one that felt all too familiar by the end of my cancer treatments.

Like most people, I had avoided pain and practised keeping it at bay by focusing on what is good and beautiful in life. I still thought that if I practised enough yoga, meditated every day, and ate the perfect foods, then I wouldn't leave any room for pain to breathe, and maybe then it would just go away and I wouldn't have to feel it anymore. Unlike birds who cannot fight against nature and eventually must emerge from their shell and learn to fly, we humans have a choice. We often choose to remain in our familiar, confining eggs and resist the urge to soar. How often do we cling to our perceived limiting ideas of what's possible, because it's all we've ever known? We fear pain as the adversary of joy and freedom, when it may actually be their midwife. Even the emotions we call negative, when approached in the right way, can help us feel what we need to heal and allow us greater access to our heart.

After radiation treatments ended, the test results came back: "positive treatment outcome." The results showed no more sign of cancer in my body. With that news, I was given the all clear. I was given my life back. In a single moment, the nightmare I had been living was over. Joy and deep relief surged through me when I heard the news, and I burst into tears. My whole body began to tremble like a wild animal who had just outrun its predator. In a huge release of adrenaline, I shook, laughed,

Chapter Five

and cried all at the same time, simultaneously overwhelmed by what had just happened, and so deeply thankful it was all over.

Although the treatments had ended and I was considered "in remission," the real healing was only just beginning. There is a difference between curing and healing. To cure is to eliminate a symptom or condition. To heal is to integrate and to make whole. You can do some deep healing and never find a cure. You can also cure something but never really heal from it.

The cancer was apparently gone, but the ravaging effects it and the challenging treatments had had on my nervous system, my psyche, and my relationships still remained. A wildfire had blazed through my life and I no longer recognized where or who I was. The body I inhabited had been transformed, both softened by motherhood and hardened by harsh treatments. The shell of my understanding had cracked, and I was now faced with the sacred task of both putting myself back together and spreading my newfound and awkward wings, unsure of where they would take me.

The twice-born yoga pose, which translates into English as the bird of paradise, symbolically implies that the paradise sought is not so much a destination, but the place of origin from which the bird came. Paradise is in the heart. It runs through her veins and powers her wings. It is the life source from which she emerges, her most natural way of being. Living in paradise is not about living in a perpetual state of bliss, unaffected by the changing tides of life. Rather it is about remembering that our natural state is one of wellbeing and wholeness. The healing we seek arises when we see all the ways we have cut ourselves off from our true nature. Remembering our innate wholeness, we can learn to accept and even welcome the pain of the breaking of the shell that encloses our understanding, and in so doing, we can make space for the unfolding of our full potential.

Salt Water Cures

The weeks that followed the end of treatments were filled with celebratory phone calls and sighs of relief. I felt like I had been given a second chance at life. I had walked through the fire and was deeply changed. Realizing how little time we have on the planet and how precious every breath is, I was clear that I want to live a life true to my soul, and I do not want to waste a single minute complaining or taking any of it for granted. I became restless with people and places that did not appreciate the preciousness of it all. As a result, some relationships and situations that had once been comfortable began to feel tight and restrictive. I struggled to squeeze into the roles I had occupied with so much ease. No longer willing to suppress my true beliefs or silence my voice, I knew that embodying my soul was what I needed to truly heal and integrate the gifts of this experience.

Shortly after treatments ended, our downtown apartment lease was up for renewal. Knowing that we would eventually need more space for our extended family, Greg and I explored where we might want to raise our child. Priced out of the expensive Vancouver real estate market, we explored our options and felt discouraged by how little we could afford (as in, nothing) in the neighbourhoods we liked. We knew we didn't want to stay in a busy urban centre, nor did we want to move out to the sprawling suburbs. We were at a loss for where to go. Remembering that we are always being supported and guided by the source of life itself, I decided to do what I had been forced to do so many times before: surrender.

When I would sit for my daily mediation practice, I'd ask for guidance to be shown the way. I would hold the question in my heart and try to relax as deeply as possible, so that I might hear or feel an intuitive nudge as to what step to take next. One

Chapter Five

morning, as I sat, I asked with my heart, "Show me where to go, where to move for the higher good of all involved." I was surprised by what came next. I felt the words "Bowen Island" appear in my mind. I had never even been to this little island before, but suggested to Greg that we go visit one day, just for fun. We decided to search for houses in our price range, and were delightfully surprised to see a few results return in our online search. We contacted the realtor of one of those houses, and arranged a visit to the island a few days later.

To our surprise, we enjoyed the twenty-minute ferry ride to the island, and liked the small-town feel of the community. Hal, the real estate agent, showed us the house we had originally come to see, then showed us another one down the street, which was also in our price range, but didn't show up in our search results because it was a foreclosure. We immediately loved the house with its wraparound porch and big back yard. The majestic cedar and pine trees that surround the property felt anchoring and healing. It had a view of the mountains and a beach nearby. Greg and I looked at each other and knew it was the one. Not knowing anyone on the island and aware of the large commitment and investment of buying our first home, we surrendered to spirit and continued to ask to be shown the next step to take. The idea of living there gave us both a feeling of excitement and lightness; in short, when we envisioned our life on Bowen Island, it felt good. Knowing that spirit speaks and offers guidance in many ways, including feelings of relief and joy, we followed the impulse and put an offer on the house. Three weeks later, we found ourselves in court.

As is the normal procedure when purchasing a foreclosed home, the hearing was to open the sale of the house to the highest interested bidder. On the morning of November 27, 2012, we got dressed for the courthouse and anxiously made our way to the hearing, with our realtor and baby in tow. Our lease at the apartment was ending on November 30. Unsure of whether we'd be awarded the house or not, three days later we would either be homeless or new homeowners. With all of the uncertainty that surrounded our house purchase, I was reminded of how little control we have on the flow of life. We can help direct the current—we can take really good care of our vessel and rig our sails—but ultimately we cannot control the wind. All we can do is be present and consciously align ourselves with the power and source of life. During that time, I kept surrendering to the outcome and asking that our next move would be clearly laid out before us.

That fateful morning in court, I anxiously bit my nails, awaiting the judge's decision on who would become the new homeowners. As she read our case out loud and announced the property value and our proposed offer, the judge asked if anyone present had a higher bid. We scanned the room nervously, hoping no one would outbid us. Not one single hand went up. With the knock of her hammer declaring it so, we bought a new house.

In hindsight, I see how much Grace played its part. In the six months that our house sat empty on the market, not a single person put an offer on it. Months after we moved to Bowen, the island experienced a boom of new families moving in, and an accompanying housing shortage. We are always shown where we need to be if we pay attention to all the ways life is speaking to us, and trust the timing of our journey.

Living among the lush trees and sprawling forest is one of the biggest draws to living on an island. After treatments ended, I wanted to get out of high-rise city living and be close to the earth. I craved nature and quiet and rest; I intuitively sensed it was what my body needed to heal.

We welcomed the quietude of island living, and appreciated the slower pace of life. But without the hustle and bustle of the

Chapter Five

city, with no loud sirens or store fronts to keep us distracted and busy, the emotional gap that lay between Greg and me came to the surface. Now that we didn't have as many appointments to use as excuses for our lack of intimacy, we realized how distant we had grown in the short time since our son was born and I had been diagnosed with cancer. I now felt like a different person; I had been transformed on a cellular level. With the gift of a second chance at life, I had little patience for excuses to live small. I sought a partner with whom to cultivate true soul intimacy; someone who would understand and accept my wild free-spiritedness and would have a similar outlook on life. I struggled to fit into the wifely role I had adopted at only twenty-five. I was no longer willing to suppress my voice and quiet my dreams to be what the world told me I should be. The idea of being a stay-at-home mom pained me; I did not want to extinguish my ambitions to travel and see the world. My desires seemed to conflict with the structure of my current life. I wasn't willing to change the circuitry of my soul or be anyone other than myself.

Arguments erupted between Greg and me like never before. The docile, pacifying, people-pleasing wife he had married no longer existed. Freed by the fire of initiation, I had emerged from the ashes like a phoenix wanting to fly. I wasn't afraid to face our issues and I could no longer force myself back into the shattered shell of my past.

A few months after we moved to the island, it became clear that I needed some solo solace time to be just with myself, grieve, and heal some of the trauma I had experienced in the year that had just passed. Greg supported my decision to take some time away from him and Ben, trusting that it was what I needed to do, to restore the sanity and loving connection we both missed between us. My parents offered to take care of our now one-year-old son, so I could go away for a week on my own.

Naturally I craved to return somewhere that nourished my soul—I packed my bags, my surf board, and my yoga mat, and headed to Costa Rica for a yoga retreat.

Awakening Desire

I arrived in Costa Rica a few days before the yoga retreat was set to begin. Friends of mine from Victoria had rented a house near Santa Teresa that week, and they invited me to stay with them until I could check into the hotel where the retreat would take place. I gratefully accepted and looked forward to connecting with friends I hadn't seen in years. Will and I had met at university in Calgary almost ten years prior. We had shared a passion for travel and spent weeks living together in Australia in our early twenties. Now engaged to his sweetheart Naomi, he had also become a yoga teacher in the years since we had seen each other, so we'd have a lot to catch up on. Since meeting Greg, I had lost touch with all of my guy friends. Will was one of those friends, and I looked forward to reconnecting with someone who had known me before the crucible of marriage, cancer, and parenthood.

When I arrived at my friends' beach house, a tall and very handsome man wearing nothing but surf shorts greeted me with a camera in his hand. As I stepped out of the cab, he helped me unload my surf board, and extended his hand to introduce himself. "Hello, I'm Gavin, a friend of Will's. I'm here taking photos for them, to promote their next yoga retreat...."

I was taken aback by his smooth South African accent and the brightness of his green eyes. He helped me carry my things into the house, and showed me to the back porch where Will and Naomi warmly greeted me with hugs and a cold beer. Even though I don't drink beer, I happily drank it that day, to

Chapter Five

quench the thirst from the six-hour drive I had just taken to get there from the airport at San Jose.

As the day went on, I enjoyed catching up with old friends, and being in the company of life-loving, free spirits. Swimming in the ocean, feeling the sun warming my skin and the saltwater washing through my short hair (which had started growing back curly), I felt myself coming back together again. I was being reborn. For the first time in years, I started to feel like myself again.

Sitting in a hammock feeling so blessed to be alive, I revelled in the sweetness of life. Somehow, I had narrowly escaped death's grasp, and here I was on the beach, feeling the warm breeze on my skin and smiling to myself, knowing how lucky I was just to be breathing. In that moment, I knew in my bones that life is truly a sacred gift, one that I would not waste trying to be anyone other than myself. Cleary Spirit still had plans for me. I still had work to do here. Watching the sunset that day, tears filled my eyes, humbled by the beauty of it all. How sad, I realized, that we often take life for granted, that we don't open the eyes of the eyes, and see the magic that surrounds us every moment of every day.

Evening came, we ate *casados* and laughed and reminisced on all the crazy adventures we had taken together. When Will lived in Australia years earlier, before I met Greg, I went to visit him while I was teaching yoga there for a few weeks. My time down under turned into a few months, after I began teaching yoga at a local studio in Noosa, Queensland. Gavin seemed fascinated by the full life I had lived during my short time on the planet. I was intrigued by his sense of wonder and amazement of it all. He was blown away that I had just gotten through cancer treatments, and didn't take his eyes off me as I spoke about what I had experienced. That evening, he invited me to go stargazing on the beach. I laughed to myself, feeling

Wildfire Within

like a giggly schoolgirl, enjoying the attention I was getting from such a handsome man. It had been years since I felt as desired as I did in that moment, and it was exhilarating. I thought I had become damaged goods. Recently bald and recovering from cancer treatments and childbirth, I never dreamed that someone would find me attractive again—I didn't even feel desired by my husband. I thought that phase of my life was over. Flirting and reawakening my sexuality was the farthest thing from my mind. I was flattered by the way Gavin looked at me and seemed genuinely interested in all that I said.

Although I wanted to go to the beach with him that night, I knew it would lead to a sandy slippery slope I might regret. I hesitantly declined, and tucked myself into bed alone, feeling revitalized after only one day in paradise. The attraction I had for Gavin was strong and it worried me. I hadn't felt this way for a man since I had met Greg. But the feeling I had with Greg was nothing like the electricity I felt coursing through my veins now. This felt so enlivening and invigorating; I was alive and, for the first time in a long time, it felt so good to be in my body again.

Over the next few days, the chemistry between Gavin and me continued to grow. He made me laugh and he thought my jokes were hilarious. He hung on every word I spoke, and made me feel radiant, beautiful, and deeply desired. We meditated on the beach in the mornings and shared our vision and dreams for life in the afternoon. When my yoga retreat began a few days later, I said goodbye to my friends at the beach house and hugged Gavin goodbye. We hadn't been physically intimate, but emotionally, we had fallen for each other. Not wanting it to be the last time we'd see each other, he promised to share the pictures he had taken once we were both back home in Vancouver on the West Coast, where he also lived.

In staying faithful to my husband that week, I felt like I was being unfaithful to myself. But I knew that if I saw Gavin again,

Chapter Five

I wouldn't be able to resist the magnetic waves of desire much longer.

Sweat It Out

The next evening, the first night of the yoga retreat, a Spanish Shaman passing through Santa Teresa invited our retreat group to participate in a sweat lodge, or *temazcal* as it's called in Spanish. Designed to create a ritual cleansing sweat, the sweat lodge has been used by indigenous peoples for thousands of years as a purification ceremony. Songs are sung and prayers offered as sweat clears the body of toxins and carries with it emotional toxins to be released. Lost parts of the soul are called back into the renewed body temple, so it can be restored and healed.

I had been in a sweat lodge years before, but this was the first time since going through cancer treatments and becoming a mother. When the sweat began, the shaman called in the four cardinal directions in Spanish and offered prayers for healing to Great Spirit. The door flap was closed, and we stayed in the domed structure until the end of the ceremony.

A fire was lit outside the lodge, where rocks were heated before being passed into the dome. Once inside, the hot rocks were carefully placed in a shallow pit then doused with herb-infused water. Steam rose from the fiery rocks and filled the tent, each time with prayers being sung, rising up to the heavens, cleansing the body and spirit. The heat intensified every time a rock was placed inside the steaming pit. When the heat became too much to bear, I lay on the cool ground and visualized the sweat dripping from my skin as though rivers of poison were pouring out of my body. Waves of nausea overcame me, and I felt myself go into a trance where I saw all the old cancer cells and chemo agents draining from my body, pulled out of me by the purifying heat of the fire. The sweat cleansed my bones and my heart.

When the beachfront ceremony ended, I crawled out of the sweat lodge along the sandy beach and went into the ocean. In the darkness of the night I swam, again feeling the water wash over me, bringing life to my newly healed cells and soul. After swimming in the ocean, I lay with my back on the beach, gazing at the moon, feeling my heart beating, enraptured by the radiance of the stars above me. In that moment, I was at one with all of life. There was nothing more to fear. I had faced death, died, and was reborn again. It is a cycle that nature knows well, and one that I will continue to meet as long as I am alive. With earth beneath and sky above, waves washed over me as I breathed air into my lungs, and felt the fire in my heart ignite, burning more brightly than ever.

Savour the Flavours

Each of the five elements (earth, water, fire, air, and space) is connected to one of our senses. Water governs our ability to taste and savour the many flavours of experience. The word *rasa* refers to the juiciness or flavours of life. For the tantric yogi, no flavour is to be left untasted. Anger, sadness, joy, fear, disgust, wonder, curiosity, and desire all add to the richness of life. If we are partial to only feeling or tasting one aspect of life, we are numbing ourselves to the full spectrum; we aren't really living to the fullest. If we only swim in the shallow waters of what we prefer in life, then we'll miss diving into the deep ocean of possibility. Like water, energy and emotions must flow to be life-giving. Stagnancy is a sort of death and so, to gain energy, we must move the energy of our watery emotions and savour every flavour.

In Ayurveda, the term *rasayana* means "rejuvenation." Literally translated as "re-juicing," it refers to the healing power

Chapter Five

of water, both inner and outer, to restore a state of vitality. It is bringing back a sense of flow, and we do it by allowing ourselves to truly feel all the emotions that flow through us, hydrating our parched soul. For water to be life-giving, it must flow. Picture a clear flowing mountain stream versus a stagnant cloudy pond. If we hold onto resentments, anger, or any unfelt emotion, the energy remains stuck in our body and blocks the natural flow of our life force. We cannot dwell in only one way of being if we are to thrive. When we allow our emotions to flow and awaken our sense of feeling, the rivers of life force within us start to move and rejuvenate our cells. A love for life and a deep enjoyment of the juiciness of being alive will naturally flow when we clear the blocks and dams we have built up inside ourselves.

By re-juicing myself with the healing salt waters of sweat, tears, and ocean waves, I felt the life force within me begin to flow again, like sweet nectar. I reconnected with the vitality of my feeling body. After a week spent sweating in the sun, the sweat lodge swimming in the ocean, and crying tears of gratitude for the gift of life, I felt rejuvenated at the deepest level. By the end of my retreat time in Costa Rica, I felt cleansed, healed, and rejuvenated. I savoured the flavour of pure effervescent joy and the bliss of being alive flowing through my veins. Water brought life back after the wildfire.

Releasing the Good Girl

I returned to Bowen Island a week later deeply rejuvenated, feeling awake to the magic of life. The feelings I had felt with Gavin stirred a passion within me that I was no longer willing to suppress. My intention, yet again, was to channel this renewed sensuality into my relationship with Greg, and hopefully breathe life back into the embers of our original spark.

When I got home, the contrast between the lives we were

both living was even more apparent. The unaffectionate tension between Greg and me grew even thicker. I wanted more emotional intimacy and suggested couples therapy. He said that he was happy and that, if I had problems with our relationship, they were my issues to figure out on my own.

He was burned out and I had a renewed thirst for life. I didn't want to dim my newly reignited light, only to meet my husband in the dark. When my attempts to repair our relationship failed, I knew I had a choice to make. No longer able to pretend as though everything was okay, and knowing that my body could no longer house lies about the unhappiness I felt in my marriage, I chose to tell Greg the truth, and revealed to him that I had fallen for someone else.

Shocked by my confession, he stepped back not knowing what to say. He placed his hand on his heart and dropped his head. As though he had just had the wind knocked out of him, he tried to catch his breath, tears streaming down his face. It was the first time I had seen Greg cry. Even during my cancer diagnosis and treatments, I never saw his stoic steadiness waver.

Relieved that he finally understood we had some healing to do together, we held each other crying, not knowing how to move forward. Greg admitted that the thought of losing me to someone else was more devastating than the thought of losing me to cancer. When the reality that I might choose another dawned on him, he finally became willing to do whatever it took to repair the rift between us. I did not want to inhibit the invigorating sensual love for life I had rediscovered with another. He did not know how to give me what I needed. After much deep prayer, many heart-to-heart discussions, and weeks of couples therapy, we decided to open our relationship.

For a month, I had a husband and a lover, and they both knew about each other. My time with Gavin awoke within me the passionate, adventurous girl I had let die when I tried to be a

Chapter Five

good Christian wife. The way Greg responded to our relational crisis caught me by surprise. He opened his mind and supported my path, and that made me feel truly loved. When I allowed out the sensual liberated woman within me and stopped trying to be the perfect wife I thought Greg wanted, the spark between us reignited.

Receive the Gift

Confused and torn between the way I felt for both men, I sought my therapist's counsel for advice. One person made me feel vibrantly alive and gorgeous in every way, the other made me feel supported and unconditionally loved. I did not want to leave my husband for another man, nor did I want to forsake my free-spirited sexy self, yet I did not want to go on being with two people; the entangled emotions were confusing and exhausting. As a tantric yogini, what I desired most was intimacy with life, with one person, through awakened monogamy. When I asked her what to do about my relationship with Gavin, she suggested, "Perhaps the gift has already been received."

The gift she was referring to was reconnecting with an abandoned part of myself; my most essential self, my soul. In my affair with Gavin, I rediscovered parts of myself I had let die—the free agent, the holy rebel, my visionary self who is untamed and here to shake things up, unwilling to settle or choose anything not aligned with her soul. The good girl who always did the right thing and was only interested in pleasing other people was no longer running the show. In fact, she died when she realized that her niceness meant shrinking and silencing her voice. Being nice only kept her small, and suppressing her truth was too painful to bear; her body would not stand for it. The vital exiled parts of myself that I had disowned and cast aside as "not me" wanted to be seen and welcomed back, reintegrated in a healthy way.

Wildfire Within

The sensual, wild, and wise woman within, the one who had been suppressed and repressed—not only in my own life but also in the lives of my mother, my grandmothers, and my female lineage for the last five thousand years—was rising up.

Holy, Healthy, Whole

The words *health* and *heal* come from the same root word meaning, "to make whole." You cannot be healthy if you deny aspects of yourself. If you are not embodying who you really are, you're not living from your wholeness, and dis-ease will develop. The whole is greater than the sum of its parts. We cannot repress the parts of ourselves we deem unacceptable or unlikable (such as our anger and our sexuality) down into the basement of our subconscious, hoping they'll just disappear, and still expect to experience vibrant health.

For the natural state of wellbeing that it's our birthright to embody, we must embrace our earthy desires and our sacred heart, our humanity and our spirituality. We are both holy and sexual beings, made of light and dark, matter and spirit, earth and sky. Radiant health happens when we remember that we contain within us the ability to taste and feel all the flavours; the full spectrum of experience. We are Divine Source learning to be human, and in the same breath, we are so much more than our humanity. We are a microcosm of the macrocosm, the image of God, the rainbow bridge between heaven and earth. The centre of our being, the heart, is where conscious earth and embodied sky converge. As above, so below.

We are told by Western religions that we are born sinful (an archery term that means "missing the mark"). In Eastern and yogic traditions, we are taught that our true nature is perfect. Perfection in Sanskrit is *purnatva*. The true meaning of the word is "wholeness." We are born perfect. Not in the sense that we are

Chapter Five

without flaw, complete, or unblemished, but that we are whole unto ourselves, full like the moon, even when she appears dark. When we remember that our true nature is perfect, it does not mean that we will never make mistakes or that we'll always be happy. It means rather that in our essence, we lack nothing. We contain the whole. We are freedom-seeking creative beings capable of making good and bad choices of hurting others and even ourselves. Which also means we are capable of unimaginable creativity, love, and healing. It is up to us to choose what we want to create.

The path of deepening intimacy in committed relationship is one where we must be willing to turn toward the darkest places within ourselves, and learn to face our shadows. It's not about picking the perfect partner or even the partner with whom you have the most chemistry, but about choosing with whom you want to do the necessary work of flowering your soul. With the cancer behind me, I could start thinking long term about my life again. When I imagined the most fulfilling relationship I dreamed of for my life, I envisioned someone who would stand by my side as my equal and be the steady river banks to my wildly divine feminine nature. with the long-view perspective of my life, it was clear that Greg was the man I wanted to spend my newly reclaimed life with.

After only a few weeks, I ended my relationship with Gavin, and Greg and I began the delicate task of rebuilding ours. The time of the dark moon, of rebirth, is symbolically a new beginning. In letting go of the limiting constraints of what we thought our marriage was supposed to look like, we let it die in a way. When we made the conscious choice of coming together again, out of the darkness of death, our relationship was reborn. Both transformed by the fires of pain, loss, and betrayal, our hearts were cracked open. From this dark place of dissolution, the spark between us was reignited.

CHAPTER SIX

Cherish the Seed: Explore Your Potential (Crescent Moon)

The Crescent Moon: Step out, mobilize, hope, have faith, reach, begin

"The journey is the gift." Sianna Sherman

"You are the one you've been waiting for." Unknown source

"Your soul knows the geography of your destiny. Your soul alone has the map of your future, therefore you can trust this indirect, oblique side of yourself. If you do, it will take you where you need to go, but more important it will teach you a kindness of rhythm in your journey." John O'Donohue

Crescent Moon

Here, the moon begins to stretch herself and awakens to a new expression, a new phase of fullness. The crescent moon represents the first fragile steps we must all take to come out of the spiritual closest and embody who we really are.

A big part of my healing journey, my return to wholeness, was reclaiming the parts of myself I had deemed unspiritual or unlovable, and learning to embrace who I really am.

Chapter Six

Somewhere along my spiritual path, I had picked up the belief that I had to perfect myself before I could be worthy of true love or everlasting happiness. I thought I had to change, make myself more worthy, or perfect my relationship with my husband, before I could experience eternal love and freedom. Subconsciously I was still looking for the Holy Grail *outside* myself, waiting for the perfect partner to complete me, looking for an enlightened teacher to show me the way to bliss. I yearned for an external healer to come along and take away all the pain and heartache that come with being human. I wanted to be free of fear and the sadness I still experienced on a daily basis, no matter how much yoga or meditation I practised.

Up until I was diagnosed with cancer, my spiritual path was a quest for happiness and perfection. A vertical climb upward, an attempt to ascend above the chaos and messiness of life to the oneness that connects us all. I was so focused on embodying the Divine that I had no idea how to embody myself. But the old scaffolding of my life had been destroyed in the wildfire. Now a mother and a cancer survivor, I was faced with the arduous task of rebuilding my life, my marriage, and myself in a way that would be aligned with whom I had become. A new life seed longed to emerge from the ashes of all that had been destroyed. No longer in pure survival mode, I could now exhale deeply, think more long term, and contemplate how I wanted to live the rest of my life.

What mattered most, now that I had just danced with death? What did I want to create with the limited time I had left on the planet? What meaning could I make out of all the madness I had lived? Now was the time to renew, rebuild, and tend to the delicate seeds of new beginnings.

When a new seed is planted in a garden, it must be

nourished with water, nutrients, and sunlight in order to grow. To nourish means to "provide the food or other substances necessary for growth." It also means to cherish, which is to protect and care for, to hold dear to your heart.

To live the liberated life I now desired to live, one that would be true to who I had become, I needed to cherish the soul force within me, and learn to treasure my innermost self. I had been transmuted by flames, initiated by fire into a new way of being in my body. No longer willing to suppress my light, silence my voice, or take anything for granted, every breath felt like a gift, another moment to savour being alive. The affair with Gavin had awakened within me not only my sexuality, but my passionate sensuality, a heightened awareness of how ecstatic it is to be embodied. By awakening to the texture of each moment, everything became miraculous. Sunlight on my skin was the most loving embrace. Rain falling on my nose was pure rejuvenation, a reminder to trust the flow of life. My son's smile was pure love, the most beautiful sight to witness.

With this new way of being in my body, the trajectory of my spiritual journey also changed. Rather than looking upward for the answers, believing that perfection was the secret to salvation and thinking that life would be better experienced somewhere else, my gaze shifted downward, to embrace all that was around me. Instead of aspiring to perfection or rushing to a completion that would never come, I began to deeply savour the journey. As I let go of outdated beliefs that I was not good enough exactly as I was in any moment, I opened instead to the newness of each breath and I discovered that spirit wasn't the only thing leading me on. The earth was guiding me too.

By *earth*, I mean all of nature: the seasons, the trees, the ocean, the butterfly, my body. The entire ecosystem of which we are a part is conscious, speaking to us and through us all the time. If we look to her, she will show us how we're meant to live. Just

Chapter Six

as the tantric yogis believe that Divine consciousness descends into finite physical form to know itself better, the sacred earth also rises to take form as human, to experience herself through us. As above, so below. Loving nature, I discovered, was not only reserved for the tree-hugging peace-loving hippies. Loving nature is ultimately about widening my embrace and learning to love myself.

Living on Bowen Island, I have become fascinated with the beauty and power of nature. Noticing giant cedars lining the streets, wild deer running through the yard, and frequent power outages due to strong winds, I became acutely aware of how disconnected our culture has become to the rhythms that govern the natural world. As much as we like to think that as humans we are above her, somehow evolved beyond the pull of the moon and the turn of the seasons, we are *of* the earth; we are expressions of nature. We will never experience vibrant health or deep fulfillment until we learn to embrace our elemental nature, to see ourselves as living vessels of the earth that sustains us. By having a spiritual practice that orients us only upward to spirit and oneness, we ignore the ground beneath us and miss the soulful uniqueness of each moment.

In many Native American and Celtic traditions, seven sacred directions are honoured to remember the totality of our being (east, south, west, north, above, below, within). Practitioners of these traditions call on these sacred directions in recognition of our wholeness and connection with all that is. We must not only look upward to heaven for spiritual connection, but all around, beneath, and within us too. We are the meeting point where all of these energies converge. The Holy Grail we seek is within the centre of our very own heart.

We are told by our culture that we must work harder and longer before we can experience success and true happiness. More is better, we're led to believe, and we could always be happier if

Wildfire Within

we were to just try the next best thing. The next diet, promotion, or lover will finally complete us and give us everything we need to experience the best that life has to offer. I was one of those people who consumed all the self-help books I could get. Under the guise of "becoming my best self," I inhaled programs and courses that promised the everlasting solution to the discomfort of my humanity. I felt guilty when I experienced "negative" feelings and, in the name of selfless service, I always put other people's needs in front of my own.

When I was diagnosed with cancer at twenty-eight years old, I realized that no amount of positive thinking could prevent pain from entering my life. Instead of eradicating sadness, I had to learn how to draw wisdom from it. Uncertainty and chaos had engulfed me like flames. Unsure of how to cope, I turned to nature to learn how to restore myself. The Great Mother, Pachamama, Madre Tierra, nature herself became my greatest teacher and guide to understanding the power and necessity of the dark.

When I moved to an island and started living among the trees in the forest, away from streetlights and sirens, I noticed how quiet and dark nighttime really is. Surrounded by the grounded presence of the trees, I sometimes slept for days at a time, feeling the healing power of deep sleep rejuvenate my bones, soothing them from the fatigue of recovering from depleting cancer treatments. The first winter we spent living on the island, I was struck by how nourishing the slower pace and inward pull of the seasons were to my soul, and how addicted I had been to the fast pace of life we had lived in the city. That state of go-go-go, constant busy-ness, and perpetual bloom that we strive to maintain as humans does not exist anywhere else in nature. Nothing is in full bloom forever. Funny, we think that we can outsmart our nature with caffeine and smartphones. When we look to nature we can see that the darkness is where all things begin.

Chapter Six

Aligning with the Moon

"The story that the moon tells is of birth, growth, fullness, decay, disappearance, with rebirth and growth again." Demetra George

Early on during my treatments, Sianna suggested I "begin syncing up with the moon." At the time, I didn't understand what she meant, until I actually started paying attention to the moon's cycles. I had never given much thought to the moonlight and was not into astrology (now I love it). But simply becoming aware of the moon's presence felt healing and in doing so, I began to dramatically shift the energy of my body.

As we know, the moon moves through phases every month. Unlike the sun yet because of the sun, she waxes and wanes, and moves toward darkness within each cycle. Her cyclic nature mirrored my own cyclic nature and reminded me of my own needs for rest and the rejuvenation of darkness. Periods of quiet and solitude are not encouraged or built into the way we live our lives, and I believe their absence leads us to burnout and the rise of chronic disease. The stress caused by trying to be only like the bright sun in the day, shining all the time, constantly plugged into productivity mode, is causing disease because it is not aligned with nature, with who we are or what we need.

We contain both the sun and the moon energies. In yoga, we have lunar and solar channels, vibrational rivers that carry both types of energy throughout our body. The solar channel is connected to the masculine principle—will, action, and liberation—what we emanate like the rays of the sun. The lunar channel is associated with the feminine—desire, our ability to feel, receive, and manifest, our radiant magnetism. Through yoga, we seek to balance the sun and the moon, the masculine and the feminine within ourself, and learn to integrate both energies into our being. It's not about either or, but the blending of both.

Wildfire Within

If we are operating in a predominantly solar way, from a goal-oriented place, always moving, achieving more, and seeking freedom, then we're not living aligned to nature. To only embody lunar energy is to become overly sensitive and moody, unable to make clear choices or take inspired action in the world. In either case, we are not embodying our wholeness. We are fragmented, only living at one end of the spectrum. Nature always seeks balance and will create the necessary wildfires and rainstorms to find its innate equilibrium.

By *balance*, I do not mean equal parts feminine and masculine all of the time. There will be times in our life when we'll be required to fan the flames of our inner sun and take courageous action in the world. Sometimes what will be needed is our moonlike ability to step back, to listen, feel, and embrace periods of apparent darkness and inactivity. True balance and real wisdom ultimately come from our ability to discern what is needed, moment-by-moment. Balance is a dynamic process, a living dance. We must be awake and present enough to feel our way into radiant wellbeing, into being well-in-one's-being.

Looking back now, I see how for many years I approached my spirituality in a very masculine or solar way. I was an avid Ashtanga yogi, practising only the primary series, a linear and progressive sequence that focused on building strength and stamina. I was rigid about the foods I ate, and I took my *sadhana* (spiritual practice) very seriously. As a type A personality, I was always trying to accomplish more, focused only on the destination, striving to reach perfection. Most of our culture is set up this way. We're told we need to do more to be complete, or that we need to buy more to experience real happiness.

For my health to return, I had to return to wholeness. I needed to embrace the whole spectrum—my humanity and my divinity—and learn to embody the fullness of who I am. I had to reawaken to the moon energy within me, the Divine

Chapter Six

femme who had been forgotten for too long. When I embarked on my spiritual journey in my late teens, I immersed myself in masculine forms of meditation and the upward pursuit of bliss. I explored consciousness and spirit and oneness, but never dove into the deep waters of my body, my unique soul, my individuality. I never considered what made me me.

After the wildfire swept through my life, a sort of darkness remained. Life had changed and I grieved the loss of innocence and simplicity of how life had been. But for the first time, the darkness I felt was not negative. The uncertainty of life, like fertile soil, was now full of potential. Out of the darkness, anything could arise. Old ways of being, diseased patterns of conformity and inauthenticity had burned away in the flames, leaving behind seeds of wisdom and desire for a new way of being to emerge. In the wake of the wildfire, I could rebirth myself and choose another way.

To truly heal and reap the gifts I had drawn from my experiences, I had to let go of trying to be perfect, and reembody the wild from which I came.

Stay Wild

The wild in you is that which is natural, creative, and wise. It is your essence, your radiant core, your soul. Your soul is the deepest part of you, that which you are here to express in this lifetime. Just as nature requires diversity and wildfires for its own sustainability and growth, the world needs you to embody your unique essence for its health and survival. We are expressions of the earth, of nature. Our growth is her growth and evolution. We often forget that we are nature. It is when we lose our connection to nature that we lose our connection to ourselves. And so we can look to nature's rhythms and patterns as guides for our own spiritual growth and unfurling soul journey.

Embracing my humanness and recalibrating to nature's rhythms have been big parts of my healing journey. Learning the language of nature inevitably transformed my perception of spirituality. As I discovered, the spiritual journey is not a smooth, upward linear trajectory. The soul's journey is a spiralling path full of curves and seeming detours. Shakti—the creative Divine feminine power of the Universe—is not one-dimensional. She twists and turns and likes to dance.

Like oceanic waves and blossoming flowers, the journey of the soul is wild and untamed, happening without our conscious will or effort. It is the inevitable journey leading us home to wholeness, to who we really are and who we're meant to become. Although you cannot stop the waves, you can try to fight the flow and waste precious life energy trying to counter the current. Or you can learn to surf and enjoy the ride of becoming who you're here to be.

As with any sport or nature-based art form such as surfing or gardening, technique and style are involved. We can learn to harness the technology to become more agile in the water or proficient with our plants. It's helpful to know where you are in relation to the waves, so you can position yourself to go with the flow and enjoy the thrill of riding them in. To understand a plant's needs, you have to learn plant language, to read the signs without talking in words, but in smells, colours, and shapes. Everyone has the ability to interpret the language of nature if they want to. Look deeper. Examine the patterns. Go with the life force.

The Circle

Very little in nature moves in a linear way; nature is cyclic—generative and destructive. Seasons fold into each other; like a great wheel, we revolve around the sun. The circle is

Chapter Six

symbolic of the feminine and of our own holistic soul journey, one that is unbroken and all-encompassing. Like nature, our human nature and soul's journey are cyclic. And like the circle and the phases of the moon, we are always whole, yet we move through different seasons of light and dark. Sometimes we feel disconnected and see only glimpses of our true nature. There are times we must let go gracefully and accept the fallow seasons between projects and places. Other times, we are called to create, produce, and radiate with fullness. We feel the joy of self-expression, and the satisfaction of knowing who we are. All are welcomed parts of the whole circle. If we are grasping onto only one part of the wheel, the ride will be clunky. If we don't honour and allow the cycles to happen, we are moving against nature. When we aren't going with the flow of life, we resist our own expansion and in so doing, we experience suffering.

To stay wild is to say yes to being alive among many other living beings, human and non-human. It is being in dynamic relationship to all of life, remembering that we are all connected and nourished by each other. Staying wild is waking up our instinctual feeling body, and remembering that our thoughts, words, and actions affect the whole. Knowing we are here to add to the beautiful diversity of creation, staying wild is to be generative, choosing ways of being that enhance life for all beings. By embracing both our earthy humanness and our unbound spirit, we can consciously create the wild we want to inhabit.

Nature's Design

In nature, things are either growing, sustaining, or dying. All three phases are happening within and around us all time. Every day, new cells within our body are forming and others are dying off. Ideas and creative projects are birthed, as relationships we've outgrown are released. Life and death are happening simultaneously. In the wild, during the deepest days of winter when all seems dark and lifeless, something new is stirring below the surface. Deep within the dark soil, a seed is breaking open, its protective skin dying essentially, dissolving so that a sprout may emerge. The essence of the seed must stretch out into the fertile soil and draw from the darkness, where it finds nourishment to grow.

One of the most potent seeds symbolizing our own soul trajectory is the humble acorn. Even as a small nut, the acorn contains within it the entire oak tree. The pattern or potential for the whole is inherent from the beginning, but the acorn must give way to radical rebirth for it to become what it's truly meant to be. Our soul is like the acorn. Unlike oaks, however, we are the only part of creation that can resist our own unfolding. Our ego's effort to remain seeds and eggs, when we're meant to blossom and soar, creates unnecessary suffering. We can either choose to remain tight buds and acorns, or give way to the fullness of who we really are. Like the acorn to the mighty oak, your soul is the spiritual blueprint for how to grow and what to become. It carries a vision, images, and desires about who you are here to be, and how your gifts serve the larger whole. Your soul's longings are not frivolous; they are helping you understand why you are here.

Eventually, after much stamina, resilience, and grace, an acorn becomes an oak tree, transforming into a source of great sustenance and beauty to many species. In the same way, our soul's evolution is part of nature's evolution; it enhances all of life on the planet. It benefits the whole and is a necessary part of the ecosystem. The world needs you to be yourself. As B.K.S. Iyengar said, "We must come to see the relationship between nature and soul; yoga does not reject one for the other but sees them as inseparably joined like earth and sky are joined on the

Chapter Six

horizon." And so we can look to nature to understand our own spiritual journey of becoming the Divine human, the embodied soul we are here to be.

As I began to pay attention to the moon and her rhythms, I learned about my own cyclic nature. Instead of pushing myself to do more or always trying to improve myself in order to perpetually shine brightly like the sun, I decided to embrace my more feminine, lunar nature. I softened into a state of receptivity, choosing to listen to my intuition about what I needed to learn, what I needed to let die, and how I could heal and grow from my walk with cancer. I surrendered to the power that governs the tides of the earth and the waters of my body: the moon.

Becoming more moonlike became key when Greg and I began the work of rebuilding our relationship from a place of authenticity and respect. In seeing the moon re-emerge from the dark and understanding her power to regenerate herself, I was given hope that our relationship could also be renewed, for it is a pattern inherent within nature. Nothing is ever wasted in nature. Garbage does not exist without the presence of humans. I knew that all the heartache we had experienced had cracked us open. From the breakdown of our relationship, we learned the power of being vulnerable with each other. No matter how difficult our relationship had been, we each had within us the potential for rebirth. As we emerged from the dark side of the moon and consciously chose to be with each other, we turned toward healing and re-wholing our relationship. During this time of the waxing light of expansion, we chose to begin again and help each other grow. By being true to who we each were, we learned how to love each other better, and we discovered what it truly means to cherish ourselves and each other.

We can work with the lunar phases over the course of a month, a year, or a lifetime. In the words of my soul sister Laura Larriva Page, "The moon can remind us that all phases and stages offer something crucial to our inner and outer development and to our connection to our essential vitality. We are, indeed, the authors of our own lives. To live full and wholehearted lives is to embrace all parts of ourselves as natural and holy. To root into the earth is to excavate and celebrate our individuality hand-in-hand with transcendence and oneness."

In whatever way we choose to move in rhythm with the moon, the lunar cycle is an integral guide of wholeness and renewal. We can look to her dynamic rhythm as symbolic of our own cyclic nature.

Be Your Own Heroine

Another wildly empowering map, which I discovered on my quest to reclaim my inner radiance, is the hero's journey. Joseph Campbell, a famous twentieth century American mythologist who is the author of *The Hero's Journey*, describes the trajectory from life's trials to triumph as "the hero's journey." In short, every hero in the making will experience and walk through these common thresholds: a separation from ordinary life, initiation through a difficult ordeal, discovery of his own true power, emergence from the underworld, and a return home bearing the gifts for his community that are born of his transformation.

This psycho-spiritual-mythical journey is the plot of every good movie, story, and novel, where the powers of light and dark battle it out until the victim becomes victorious. As humans, we love this story, because it speaks to the hero within each of us; the one inside who is courageous, resilient, and here to serve.

Not long after Joseph Campbell released his work into the world, a few female students felt it didn't accurately describe their experience as women. The journey they had lived was more nuanced, one of separation from and reintegration with

Chapter Six

self. A long-time student of Campbell's, Maureen Murdock, charted an alternative path to the hero's journey, one she believes to be more descriptive of the feminine journey to the underworld. *The Heroine's Journey*, aligning with Murdock's model, is divided into ten stages. Below is my interpretation of the Murdock heroine journey:

The Heroine Separates from the Feminine

When we lose touch with the sacred feminine, our heroine's journey begins.

Often as a mother or in a societally prescribed feminine role, we reject the feminine within ourselves.

The Heroine Identifies with the Masculine and Gathers Allies for a New Way of Life

This often requires that the heroine choose a path that is different from the limiting roles prescribed for her. This is when she tries to make it in a man's world, by becoming more like a man; for instance, she climbs the corporate ladder in a patriarchal system to prove that she is capable.

The Heroine Faces Her Demons and Fears

The heroine encounters the inner and outer demons of self-doubt, limiting beliefs, and people who try to keep her small.

The Heroine Experiences Success by Society's Standards

By overcoming obstacles, she is given a taste of success. This would typically be where the hero's tale ends. The heroine has more to do.

The Heroine Awakens and Feels Spiritually Dead

Success in this new way of life is not all it's cracked up to be. It feels too limited, temporary, illusory, shallow, and requires a betrayal of self over time.

The Heroine Receives an Initiation and a Descent into the Goddess

The heroine faces a crisis of some sort, in which the new way is insufficient and falls into despair. All of her "masculine" strategies have failed her.

The Heroine Urgently Yearns to Reconnect with the Feminine

She feels the need for her femininity, but cannot go back to her initial limited way of being in the world.

The Heroine Heals the Mother/Daughter Split

She reclaims her sacred feminine values and sees them as gifts of her empowerment.

The Heroine Heals the Wounded Masculine Within

The heroine makes peace with the "masculine" approach to the world as it applies to herself, and she understands how it has served her. Her journey is not about the feminine over the masculine, but about learning to integrate both.

Chapter Six

The Heroine Integrates the Masculine and Feminine

She understands the need for both the sacred masculine and the sacred feminine, and learns how to embrace both aspects of herself and live from a place of wholeness.

My path to healing was my own heroine's journey, a return to wholeness, to true integration of all parts of myself.

In my own life, I separated from the sacred feminine in my late teens, when I adopted a spirituality that led me on a quest for perfection. I became really good at suppressing my feelings and achieving all my goals in an attempt to find happiness. I would try to override my deep anger or sadness with positivity, always reaching for the light. But when I was diagnosed with cancer, my positive spirituality felt like a bubble-gum view of reality. It was not big enough to contain the fullness of my experience. I had to turn toward the darkness, the discomfort of thinking about my own death, and learn to embrace paradox. I looked to nature, the Great Mother, and to more feminine versions of spirituality to reclaim what I had denied in myself for too long: my body, my soul, my fragile humanity. The integration of the masculine and the feminine within myself was the remembrance and full embrace of my eternal sacred spirit, and the holiness of my flesh, the earth, and this moment.

The Five Layers: Your Five Bodies

The heroine's journey is essentially a journey to the centre of our being, to our innermost self. Intuitively sensing this innate sacred centre, ancient yogis journeyed from the outer physical body layer to the innermost subtle soul layer. Through meditation, yoga, and breathing techniques, they discovered there is indeed more to this "being human" thing than meets the eye. Moving from the outside in, they unearthed a five-layered model to describe the journey from the outermost layer of our body to the soul gold within.

The five sheaths (or *pancha koshas* in Sanskrit) are our five bodies, creating an anatomical map guiding us on an inward journey from the outermost layer of our physical body to the more subtle yet influential layers of energy, emotions, wisdom, and soul.

Physical Body

The physical body is *annamaya kosha* in Sanskrit. Literally translated as "food body," this is our outermost physical layer. All that we can see with the eyes, it is made of bones, blood, organs, muscles, and skin.

Energy Body

Our energy body is made of our vital life force. It's the part of us that feels tired or energized; it reflects our level of vitality. *Prana* is Sanskrit for "life force," and so this is our *pranamaya kosha*.

Emotional-Mental Body

Our thoughts, feelings, and emotions make up our emotional body, or *manamaya kosha* in Sanskrit. Translated as the "mind-heart body," this is the part of us that feels all the feelings, the fluctuation of energy known in the form of thoughts and emotions.

Intuition Body

This is the deeper wisdom within us, the intuitive part of the

Chapter Six

self that is connected to higher knowing. *Vijnanamaya kosha* in Sanskrit is the inner knowing that can be trusted without explanation.

Bliss Body

The Golden Buddha within, this is the treasure buried as the innermost self. Known as the *anandamaya kosha* in Sanskrit or "bliss body," this is the centre, the core, the essence of who you are. Your true nature is made of joy and love. More profound than happiness, the bliss body is described as the joy of being alive. Joy and love feel so good in our bodies because they are the most closely aligned with our true nature.

Although none of these layers is really separate from the others, we can think of them like *matryoshka* dolls (the wooden nestling Russian dolls) that bring us closer to the centre as we remove each layer. The difference, however, is that instead of getting smaller the closer we get to the core, the more subtle layers are the most pervasive, meaning that they have a greater outward reach. The innermost self, the bliss of the soul, is the brightest and most influential, radiating out through all the other layers. When we remember that we are a soul having a human experience, all of the outer layers of our being come into greater harmony and balance. In other words, our soul is the most powerful and affective part of our self; when we connect to our soul, it ripples throughout and recalibrates all the other parts of our being, creating greater vitality. We must nourish all of our bodies—the physical, psychological, emotional, and spiritual—and the more we are aware of the deeper unseen layers and work from the inside out, the better we'll feel on all levels.

Remembering that we are so much more than what we see is also a useful reminder when we are feeling lost or sorry for ourselves. If we only identify with one layer of our being, we suffer. If we think we are only a body, then we'll inevitably feel sorrow when we age or become ill. If we are overly identified with our energy body or our emotional-mental body, then we'll mistake our lethargy or sadness for who we really are. We'll believe everything we think about ourself.

The beauty of seeing our five layers of being is that we remember that we are so much more than our physical body, our energy levels, our thoughts, and our desires. Our freedom lies in choosing to stay connected to our centre, aligned to who we really are as a soul, so we can emit an inner light outward, back out through all the other layers. We can be the lighthouse and choose to shine, rather than let the external storms extinguish our inner flame.

That healthy glow that we all seek is not a result of using the right moisturizer or thinking only happy thoughts. It comes from knowing who we are, and allowing that knowledge to pour into our whole life, through all of our bodies. Although the five sheaths are described like Russian nestling dolls layered on top of each other, they are not separable, like the wooden dolls are. You cannot take off your physical meat suit to reveal your energy body, or strip your mind down to don only your soul body. There is no place where your spirit ends and your mind begins, or where your mind ends and your body begins. Our body-mind-soul is a continuum of energy, not separate parts that we need to join together through mindfulness, but a spectrum of vibration.

Often in religious circles, the body is seen as "less spiritual than" or not as sacred as the soul. But in reality, the body is an expression of the soul, an outer manifestation of a Divine source. The physical body is the outermost and densest aspect of who we are, but it is no less holy than the soul. If anything, the body is what allows us to experience this life in all its glory.

Chapter Six

It is not only the vehicle for our soul-force, but the very means by which we can know ourselves.

Your Body is the Living Vessel

For this reason, the body is often described as the temple. Yes, it is a temple because within it dwells a sacred presence. But anywhere we find ourselves can become a place of worship, if we remember the holy source from which we all emerge. For the awakened soul, the body is the temple, but so is the kitchen, the car, the workplace, the bedroom. The temple is everywhere. It is where the power of our presence meets the sacredness of each moment.

Although I like the imagery of the body as a temple, I prefer to think of the body as a living vessel that responds to how we inhabit it. We are like potters, moulding our physicality through focus and attention. The body is not static—it is ever changing, renewing itself, always responding to the more subtle bodies within it. The body is like a clay dwelling, always reshaping itself according to our beliefs and choices. The fires of life are like the kiln that serves to strengthen and solidify who we are.

From a yogic perspective, energy flows from invisible to visible. The most subtle body (the bliss body or soul) has the greatest influence on all the other bodies. Just as a pebble dropped in water ripples outward creating changes on the surface of the lake, our most visible body (our physical body) responds and vibrates to what is happening at the centre. It is easier and more effective to create change by going straight to the source, to drink from the inner wellspring of love and to remember that within every beautiful body is a soul here only to bloom.

Being healthy means being whole and living with all of your bodies integrated. If we only identify as a body and neglect the care of the soul, we will inevitably suffer as we age or fall ill. Remembering that we are so much more than a body and knowing that our body responds to not only the mind but, more importantly, to our innermost soul self will keep us anchored in the centre of who we are.

When I was diagnosed with cancer, a wave of anger and distrust came over me. How could my body betray me like this, after I had taken such good care of it, I thought? Wasn't all the yoga and healthy food supposed to protect me from getting a terminal illness? What I did not understand at the time was that working from the outside in will only get you so far. If you're drinking green juices and exercising, your body will naturally respond; you'll have more energy and you'll feel better than if you weren't doing those things. But true health happens when we are deeply rooted in the knowing that we are each on a heroic soul journey, here to shape matter and share our sacred spark.

During my early treatments, I did not appear to be sick. From the outside, I looked okay. Eventually, I started losing weight and all my hair. I'd wear wigs to conceal my condition, but I knew they weren't addressing what was happening inside. They were only serving to cover it up. Living by caring only for the physical is like trying to heal cancer by wearing a wig. As ridiculous as it sounds, we do this all the time when we see ourselves only from the outer layer of our physical body. We can change what we wear or who we sleep with, but it won't get to the root of what we really need. It's like rearranging the living room furniture while the house is burning down.

In my darkest days, no matter how much I wanted to run away or live someone else's life, it finally dawned on me that there was nowhere I could go that my cancer was not. I carried it inside me. Even more terrifying (or reassuring, depending on the day) was that there was nowhere I could travel where I was not. I could try to run from my problems and my marriage; I could attempt to numb the pain and cover up my cancer with

Chapter Six

fancy hairpieces; but I could never escape the relationship I had with myself.

If I wanted to heal and see the outer circumstances of my life change, I'd have to start with loving myself, exactly as I was, from the inside out. From the level of soul, I needed to embrace who I am and trust that my body's innate wisdom would recalibrate to the stream of love that would begin to flow through my veins. I had to re-member, literally put myself back together, starting by cultivating an intimate relationship with my innermost self.

My soul, or bliss body, the essence of me, communicates to my physical body via the language of emotions, thoughts, and intuition. Cancer wasn't who I am. It was a disruption on my outermost layer, an engine warning light signalling me to stop and pay attention to what was happening inside.

So often we look outside ourselves to understand who we are. We allow the job, the lover, or the wrinkles to define our capacity to love ourself. We imagine that after losing that last five pounds, after the next big launch, or after the victory we'll have the key to ensure our lifelong happiness. But the five bodies show us that there is another way to access the deep joy we all want.

Instead of looking outward to quench our thirst for bliss, we can drink straight from the wellspring of self-knowledge. By seeing ourself as a soul on a heroine's journey, here to reveal the unique radiance that is solely ours to embody, we can reclaim our place as sacred co-creators on the material plane and see our life as a creative act.

Rather than thinking of myself as a sickly cancer patient, I chose to look at my cancer as a messenger, a manifestation of miscommunication. I knew that I am a soul having a human experience, but even then, I didn't really embrace who I am, or know how to embody that deeper part of me. Instead, I tried to be spiritual, the way other people are spiritual, in an effort to know God. In other words, I was looking for love in all the wrong places, outside myself and my present-moment experience. I thought I had to change the outer manifestation before I could be free of the cancer. But it was only once I recalibrated myself to my soul nature, that my body began to heal.

For power to flow into a light bulb, the electrical wire needs to be grounded to the earth or a stabilizing force. Only then can the light shine brightly. For our own inner radiance to flow, we need to embrace all our bodies as one continuum, an expression of our sacred source. If we are not grounded, both plugged into who we are on the level of soul and rooted in our body and the earth, then we risk becoming depleted or burnt out. We can only shine our light when we're anchored into the true source of who we are.

Our intuition body is the way our light or bliss body communicates to us, through our thoughts, emotions, and bodily sensations. It's important to trust your intuitive impulses, for they are direct messages from your soul. Your innate guidance system is there to help you make choices that will allow your soul's gifts to really develop and be offered through the way you live your life. The way of your soul is wild; you did not come here to walk along a well-charted path and to be like everyone else. The soul of you is here to blaze its own trail. Yet it is very wise and will always lead you toward your greatest good, toward that which will allow its full expression through your life.

We are each on a spiritual journey, our own heroine's quest, whether we are aware of it or not. Life is full of challenges, trials, and pain. There's no getting around that. But it is how we choose to relate to our pain, how we engage with the tribulations, that will awaken our capacity for healing and wholeness.

We are the one we've been waiting for. The hero or shero we long for is within our own heart. She is the radiant one within who is strengthened by pressure and heat. Like a diamond, she

Chapter Six

is the one who becomes fortified and more sure of who she is with every passing struggle. Through life's hardships, she remains centred, and becomes more clear, strong, and vibrant with every passing day, bringing her soul beauty to the world.

As we consciously choose how to view and how to engage with the inevitable struggles of life, we embark on the soul's journey of becoming our own heroine.

May we remember that we are each a heroine in the making. Our life *is* our heroine's journey and the gift is the journey itself.

Don't Mistake the Map for the Journey

Of course, we can never mistake maps for the territory. Mistaking the tiny finger pointing at the moon for the moon itself will fall short of witnessing the full moon illuminate the night sky. Learning about Paris and tasting a warm buttery croissant melt on your tongue in a Parisian café are two totally different experiences. The soul's journey—and, of course, life—is not a defined path that can be described or hacked by studying a map. We are each blazing our own trail as we go. We get to write our own story. But the maps that we come across along the way can help us savour the calm seasons, channel our creativity, and navigate the stormy waters that inevitably come. They can serve as guideposts and beacons, shining a light on how we can maximize the gifts of our journey and make the most of our time here.

When you find yourself in the dark night of the soul, may you take heart, trusting that you are there to be strengthened, shaped, and ensouled. May the growing light of the crescent moon instil within you the courage to have faith and begin anew. May you cultivate a deep knowingness of who you are, a stability deep inside your bones, so that the vitality, clarity, wisdom, and bliss of your true self can step out and shine through.

Wildfire Within

Sacred maps can serve to remind us of the bigger picture, so that we may remember that night is always darkest before the dawn, the new moon always move toward fullness, and the soul, like a diamond, always becomes more radiant through the wildfires of life.

CHAPTER SEVEN

Nourish the Root: Nurture Your Nature (First Quarter Moon)

First Quarter: Activate, build, risk, be confident, plunge in, promise, commit

"My soul is dying to be free. I can't live the rest of my life so guarded. It's dying to be free. It's up to me, to choose what kind of life I lead." Marié Digby, *"Unfold"*

"The most authentic thing about us is our capacity to create, to overcome, to endure, to transform, to love and to be greater than our suffering." Ben Okri

First Quarter Moon

As the moon expands toward fullness, she widens her embrace and grows in light through the First Quarter Moon. Symbolically this phase of the moon represents our ability to make clear choices toward that which we want to create in the world and to follow through on our value-aligned decisions with action. This is the part of the heroine's journey after we've emerged from the underworld, have gone through the fire of transformation, and are ready to bring forth the gifts we have gathered from our experience.

Becoming a Conscious Creator

"You were created to create." John O'Donohue

The core of who we are, the soul, is directly connected to Spirit. Within us, the Divine dwells in us, as us. We are each God/Goddess, experiencing the world through the life of Chantal or Julie. As such, our nature as Divine beings means not only that we are sacred, but that we are also here to create.

Through the tantric lens, God/Goddess is not sitting outside her creation, judging how the whole things has gone astray. Goddess continues to create through us. God is not a finished product. *You* are not a finished product; you are continually creating your life on a daily basis, whether you are consciously aware of it or not.

Having been a big believer in *The Secret* by Rhonda Byrne and the law of attraction before my cancer diagnosis, I thought everyone created their own reality, and was responsible for the fruit they bore or the mess they made. A big shadow side of this worldview is that we can judge others or ourselves when we create undesirable life conditions. I struggled with this when I was first diagnosed, wondering how I had manifested cancer. Why would I create this? I was embarrassed and ashamed that somehow, I hadn't mastered the law of attraction, and in fact created something terrible. Layered on top of the anger of my diagnosis was a feeling of guilt that somehow I had messed up; I had created a crisis because of my sloppy thinking habits or negative vibrations.

It is true that we are creating our reality to some extent, but so is everyone else. And although we have agency as to how we manage our life force, ultimately, we don't have control over what life throws our way. What we do have agency over, however, is our experience of reality: the way we choose to view

Chapter Seven

the circumstances of our life and how we respond to the various wildfires we'll be transformed by during our time here. As such, it's not so much that we create our own reality, but more that we are always co-creating it. Whether we're conscious of it or not, we are collaborating with Spirit and other co-creators all the time. We cannot create without either. We cannot know ourself through ourself alone. It is only through relationship that we can really know ourself and become who we're meant to be. A single thread woven on a loom cannot understand or live out its purpose on its own. It alone cannot stretch itself enough to create a tapestry. It is only by weaving itself with other threads that it can understand its place, and contribute to the unfolding of the whole. We cannot know what the finished piece will look like; we have no way of knowing the final outcome. But what we can influence, we must. It's not about controlling the conditions, but about consciously choosing what we make of them. As expressions of an innately creative Universe, we are here to create. We are each responsible for the way we weave our own individual thread into the great tapestry of life.

Be a Creator, Not a Reactor

We each need to become more energetically responsible. On a soul level, we are creative beings. Like God/Goddess/The Universe, our soul is not a fixed entity finished and complete, but the essence of who we are. Our core nature, like the source from which we spring, is creative and always in a state of flow. It is in that state of both being and becoming at the same time; the living paradox of being whole as you are, yet always moving toward expansion.

Because water is always moving, it is said that you cannot step into the same river twice. In the same way, Source is always flowing to you and through you. We need only feel into the current our soul wants to take us, be present enough to hear the still small voice inside, and pay attention to what the sacred wants to create through us.

As humans made of earth and sky, bodies and souls, we are wired to be both reactors and creators. Literally, our wiring—our nervous system—is like two wings connected by a see-saw. One wing is the parasympathetic nervous system (PNS), which is the rest-and-digest response that takes over when you are in a relaxed state, able to contemplate, meditate, and assimilate. It's the space from which we can dream and vision and have big ideas. The other wing is the sympathetic nervous system (SNS), the fight-or-flight-or-freeze response that makes you want to quit things (flight) or blame other people (fight) when things don't go the way you want. It's also the part of you that will get things done, the part that will get fired up for a good reason, and inspire passion and enthusiasm for change. When one is up, the other is down. The key is knowing when to move from one to the other.

We need both, that's why we have both. It's not about being in a state of perpetual bliss, where we'll never be triggered or stressed again. It's about creating balance, and being intentional about where, inside ourselves, we spend our time. It goes without saying, that most of us spend so much time in fight-or-flight mode (reacting to what he said, worrying about what she'll think, dealing with short-term crises), that we forget there is another way to inhabit our bodies and our lives.

Yoga sees the nervous system as the medium through which the emotional-mental body communicates with the physical body. The nervous system responds to what's on your mind and carries its messages via the energy body throughout the physical body. This means that whatever you're thinking about is sending messages absorbed by your physical body and triggering one of two responses: react (stress hormones pump through blood,

Chapter Seven

deal with crisis, let outside circumstances govern direction) or create (build immunity, intentional mood, envision long-term projects).

The more we learn to inhabit the creator part of ourselves and awaken our inner artist, the more our life will become a work of art, and the fewer will be the things we have to react to. Because we are born natural creators, creating is where our true power lies.

Soul and Spirit

Perhaps you are wondering by now if there's a difference between spirit and soul. These terms are used interchangeably, but refer to very distinct aspects of our spiritual journey.

Spirit is the universal oneness that connects us all. *Soul* is your essential nature and what makes you different from anyone else. Your soul is what Bill Plotkin describes as the unique gift you carry for others or what is genuinely yours to offer the world. Spirit is the knowing that at the most fundamental level, all is well. "The soul tenaciously, constantly, and ferociously *gives a shit*," as Elisa Romeo says in *Meet Your Soul*. Spirit is coming home to the steady source of Universal love that is eternally there for us. Soul invites us to the fulfillment of playing our unique part in the whole of creation. Spirit is like the Sun, consistently steady, masculine, always shining. The soul is like the moon, deep and mysterious, feminine, cyclic, always taking a more circuitous road. Spirit is Oneness.. Soul is You-ness.

Early on in my spiritual quest, I didn't realize there was a difference, nor did I have any concept of why it would matter. But as my heroine soul's journey started to unfold, and my spiritual beliefs unraveled before my eyes, I questioned the purpose of my piousness. If the years spent on my yoga mat meditating and praying my problems away didn't safeguard me from pain and grant me God's favourable attention, perhaps I was looking for God in all the wrong places. Instead of trying to become more spiritual or pure, my cancer wakeup call was asking me to become more human, more myself. Life didn't need another perfected being, walking around in a state of perpetual bliss. Life was asking me to consciously integrate and embody my soul, the only one I was born to be.

Nourish Your Soul

As important as it is to feed and nourish our physical body, even more importantly, I believe, is that we tend to and nourish our soul, our bliss body. Plants have a major root called a taproot, from which other, smaller roots sprout outward. Because our soul is the deepest layer of our being, we can think of it as the taproot that sustains and nurtures all the other layers. Our intuition, emotional-mental, energetic, and physical bodies are all supported and upheld by the health of our soul body. If the taproot is strong, if the soul is nourished, then its radiance ripples outward, causing the inevitable flourishing of our lives.

Soul is what is most wild and natural within us. It is deeply connected to the natural world, and thus is nourished by being in nature. Just as our body loves healthy food and exercise, our soul loves nature and beauty. The soul is the part of us that finds things to be beautiful. When we follow beauty, we follow what feels alive, inspiring, nourishing, and compelling. We can then learn how to nourish ourself on the deepest level.

For reasons unknown to me at the time, when my cancer treatments were over, I deeply craved to be in nature. Little did I know when we moved to our island home in the forest that it was my soul longing to immerse herself in the rejuvenating power of the wild. Witnessing the beauty of the turning seasons, I was reminded of my own cyclic way of being in the world. Beholding

Chapter Seven

the gorgeous earthy presence of the rugged Coast Mountains, feeling the ocean waves wash over my skin, and filling my lungs with the energizing West Coast air, I immersed myself in the elements. Nature helped me heal by becoming whole again. By remembering that I too am made of earth, water, fire, and air, my cells recalibrated to my most essential self. I rediscovered within me a new kind of fire, one that is wild and creative, burning with a love for life, here to shine brightly in a uniquely specific way.

Become Soul-Centric

Being selfish in our culture has been given a bad reputation. We (especially we women) are taught to put other people's needs first and to tend to ourselves last, once we've done everything else on our long to-do list. Self-care is seen as indulgent, a narcissistic luxury for those who are needy and high maintenance. We need to turn this notion inside out: self-love and self-care are not selfish. As Danielle LaPorte says, being selfish is a Divine responsibility, and self-care is part of our spiritual practice. Tending to your own soul flame is the most loving thing you can do for others.

In my twenties I travelled the world reminding people to don their own oxygen mask first, before helping others. Then I became a yoga teacher and forgot this beneficial safety instruction that is not only useful for air travel. I started to believe that by saying yes to everyone who needed my help and working overtime to accomplish my SMART (Specific, Measurable, Agreed-upon, Realistic, Time-based) goals, I was on the fast track to spiritual enlightenment. Often exhausted and never feeling quite good enough exactly as I was, I overrode my body's cues for rest with some positive thinking and caffeine. I thought selfless service was about giving of myself and only focusing on the good of others. I ignored the reciprocity that is necessary for optimal flow and, over time, I depleted my life force.

Well, no need to reiterate how that turned out! Not only did my body shut down in an effort to get my attention, but in so doing, I became unable to help people in the only way I knew how: by over-giving myself. Suddenly, I had to rely on other people to support and serve me, and I was forced to learn how to deeply receive. For a perfectionist type A spiritual seeker, asking for help and accepting it was one of the hardest things to do. As an exhausted new mama with very limited free time and energy, I had to learn to set boundaries and be okay with disappointing people. Resting, sleeping, and minimizing stress meant that I had to get really clear on what was helping me heal and what was hindering my health. As I began to listen to the whispers of my soul and act on where my intuition was guiding me, I developed the courage to say no, unapologetically, when my heart wasn't aligned with what was being asked of me. I knew that for my physical body to heal and thrive again, I had to cherish and nourish my soul body first.

We are the ones responsible for cultivating the unique gift we each carry, and for the energy we bring out into the world. Taking time to read, travel, bathe, and write are not idle pastimes if they allow you to spend quality time with your deepest self. Nourishing your soul is following your particular beauty way, noticing what inspires you, and letting your joy, rather than your fear, lead the way. We must learn to see our self-care not as an egotistical pursuit, but as essential to our wellbeing. To be self-centred is to only think of yourself. To be soul-centric is to recognize that it is only from a place of wholeness and health that you can contribute to the greater good. Your *sadhana*—your spiritual practice—is not selfish; it is your sacred duty to keep your inner wild fire burning.

To nourish the root of who you are, to nurture your nature,

Chapter Seven

is to cherish the unique soul force within you. It is fanning the flames of what ignites your joy for life, and trusting the embers that spark within you the remembrance that beauty knows the way home. Nurturing your nature is seeing yourself as a soul embodied, a freedom-seeking creative being here to joyfully blend spirit and matter. It is about loving being and becoming you, the only you that ever was or will be. Ultimately, to nurture your nature is to reveal your soul's radiance and let the wildfire within you shine.

CHAPTER EIGHT

Tend to the Shoot: Embody Freedom (Gibbous Moon)

Gibbous Moon: Clarify, persevere, ask, design, progress, expand

"Everything can be taken from a man but one thing, the last of human freedoms: to choose one's own attitude in any given set of circumstances—to choose one's own way." Viktor Frankl

"Wherever you stand, be the soul of that place." Rumi

"Beauty begins the moment you decide to be yourself." Coco Chanel

"Protect your heart so that you can keep it wide open." Danielle LaPorte

"Freedom is the capacity to become who we truly are." Nietzsche

Gibbous Moon

As the waxing moon's light expands toward fullness through the Gibbous Moon, here she refines her raw power and clears away anything keeping her from blooming fully. *Gibbous*

Chapter Eight

means "bulging," and like a pregnant woman about to give birth, the energy of this phase is full of potential. It is also a time when stamina and discernment are required to cut away the excess and clear the schedule of what no longer serves, making space for life to blossom.

Vibrant Health

Freedom has been something I've always sought and valued. For years, I believed that freedom meant being able to do whatever I wanted, whenever I wanted. It was about having no limitations, I thought, nothing holding me back from living the life of my dreams.

With this idea of freedom in mind, I felt restrained when I became a wife, a new mother, and as someone living with a cancer diagnosis. I thought that because of all these "restrictions and conditions," I could not truly be free to be or do what I wanted. With this skewed perception of liberation, I subconsciously stifled myself, dimming my inner light and postponing my effervescent joy until the promise of some future event would set me free. Believing that I couldn't truly be free until my child was grown or my cancer cured, I felt trapped in the circumstances of my life.

It wasn't until I rediscovered the Sanskrit word for health that I realized I was the only one keeping myself captive. No one was placing limitations on my freedom but me. *Svastha* is the Sanskrit word for health. Literally translated as "seated in the self" or "established in the soul," this word implies that health comes from being who we really are. The wellbeing we all seek comes from "being well in one's being," from enjoying being yourself and embodying your unique, sacred soul. It doesn't matter how much you exercise or detox, if you don't know who you are in your core. To be healthy is to be rooted in the knowing that you are a unique being, here to embody who only you can be. It's not about being perfect or free of afflictions. It's about being whole—wholly holy you.

This idea was revolutionary for me. I realized that for as long as I could remember, I was trying to be healthy by consuming all the externals that promised to free me of bodily pain and suffering. I was "doing all the right things," such as eating a plant-based diet, teaching yoga, and doing what I loved, but it was still with the underlying vibe that only once I reached X (insert "advanced yoga pose," "perfect abs," "money in the bank," "followers on a social") would I be truly free. By trying to control life's circumstances, I was trying to create freedom from the outside in. When my failed attempts at health didn't work (enter cancer), I was forced to uncover the true meaning of "being seated in the soul."

All this is not to say that I believe I created my cancer, or that somehow my aims at living a healthy life were for the wrong reasons. We are each on our own journey and I believe we are given exactly what we need along the way to grow and evolve into who we're meant to be in the world. For me, cancer was not an invitation to eat better or even change my lifestyle in any drastic way. My cancer encounter was a wakeup call to heal the relationship I had with myself. It was an initiation into the fertile darkness, the feminine, where all life begins; a destined crossroad where I was to meet my own soul, the essence of me, and discover what truly nourishes her.

Of course, taking care of ourselves on the physical level is deeply important, as we know that our body is made of the food we eat. Developing healthy habits are key to creating lasting vitality. Regular sleep, exercise, and healthy relationships are necessary components of living a healthy life. But if we are only approaching our health from the exterior, from our outermost layers of our physical, energetic, and emotional-mental bodies,

Chapter Eight

then we'll miss the opportunity to draw from a deeper wellspring, a source far more powerful in its ability to affect the body and create the positive changes in our life and in the world that we all seek. True wealth and health comes first from nurturing the relationship we have with our innermost self.

Grow Roots and Wings

If knowing and taking care of ourself on the level of soul is so important, what is it exactly that nourishes the soul?

As we are each unique in our own soul constellation of desires, destiny, and gifts, there is not a one-size-fits-all approach to nourishing our true nature. But just as there are certain foods that promote health in the body, there are certain nutrients that provide fuel for our soul's expansion.

Common elements that sustain the soul are the elements themselves. Nature has a way of recalibrating us from the inside out. When we immerse ourselves in the beauty of the natural world, we are reminded from where we come: a place of seasons, cycles, and diversity. Nothing is wasted in nature and everything is needed. The waste from one creature gives nutrients to roots of the trees. The fallen leaves serve as building materials for the birds' nests and homes. The purifying exhale of plants is cycled back into our oxygenating inhale.

In the same way, every part of our life, every moment of our soul's journey contains within it exactly what we need to grow in the way we are meant to—if we choose to view it as such. Even the difficulties we experience can become food for the soul, powerful fertilizers sprouting us into wholeness.

When a wildfire blazes through a forest, diseased trees are destroyed, along with the old healthy trees. In the wake of the flames, the nutrients found deep within the barks and leaves of the healthier trees are released back into the earth. For some species of plants, the heat of the fire is what's needed to crack open their otherwise dormant seeds. The fire unlocks the potential for new growth, by providing heat, friction, and nourishment for new trees to sprout. When a life threatening dis-ease swept through my own life, I was forced to let go of everything I thought I was: the healthy yogi, the good girl, the perfect wife; they were all destroyed in the fire.

What remained after all my self-created identities (my ego) went up in flames was the one within me who is here to live. My most raw, real, and essential self that longs to be known and expressed. Feisty, fiery, and full of passion, she wants to be seen, felt, and known. It was time to tend to wild soul fire within me, forgotten, ignored, and repressed for too long. My cancer crisis became the catalyst to liberate the light within me, my soul, the one I had sanitized and suffocated by trying to be spiritual and good.

If we ignore our soul for too long, times of darkness are sometimes necessary to awaken us to her needs. When we live in a way that denies the soul's existence, she will do what she must to get our attention. Not to punish or hurt us, but to liberate us from our own limiting beliefs. The epidemic levels of depression, anxiety, and addiction that we're experiencing as culture, I believe, are because we've ignored tending to our souls for far too long.

Considered "maladies of the soul" in some cultures, anxiety and depression are not issues that will go away by popping pills or thinking happy thoughts. The state of our world with its tense political climate and heating environmental crisis are all symptoms of a deeper dis-ease, a discomfort we all feel when we're not aligned with who we are on the soul level. By placing economic growth as the goal of all we do, we've forgotten that there is more to life than getting rich and accumulating bigger and better things. We've ignored the earth, our outermost

Chapter Eight

body, and our soul, our innermost self. In denying the natural rhythms that govern the tides and the seasons, we're living out of alignment with who we really are; it's no wonder chronic disease continues to rise. As Bill Plotkin says "the egocentric society cuts out its own heart and attempts to live without it." By disconnecting from nature and our own soul, we've cut ourselves off from the source of life. Vibrant health and deep fulfillment cannot be acquired by producing and consuming more stuff. In nature, times of darkness (new moon, night time, deep winter) are also the most rejuvenating. To find the light, we must honour, embrace, and welcome the dark.

The dark that I speak of here is not an evil force, although it has been demonized by patriarchy, because it is so little understood. It is not the opposite of good, as in good versus evil and light versus dark. The dark is how the Great Mystery shapes us into who we're here to be. Like the womb, the dark is a deeply nurturing and creative space. Pregnant with potential, the "dark night of the soul" is where anything becomes possible. When old structures break down, energy is released, free to move in ways that are new and healing. Times of crisis are also times of wild creativity. The Chinese character for "danger" is also the same symbol for "opportunity."

In nature, everything begins in the dark. When things are falling apart, something new is being born. Visualize the seed breaking through its membrane to form roots and shoots; or visualize the rejuvenation of deep winter. The winter solstice, the darkest part of the year is also when we celebrate the return of the light. Like the daylight, the springtime, and our own embryonic origin, everything beautiful and good emerges from the dark. I've become so attuned to the rhythms of nature and my soul's creativity that I now welcome times of seeming inertia and decay; I trust the cycle and power of transformation, knowing that something new below the surface is being churned.

Metamorphosis can be frightening. When we're in the dark womblike cocoon spaces of radical transmutation, we don't know what to expect. But times of uncertainty can also be deeply exhilarating. They remind us that we are alive, and that the nature of life is change. When the caterpillar instinctively weaves itself into a cocoon, transitional or imaginal cells begin the process of digesting the caterpillar's body, and then secrete the genetic blueprint for the immanent butterfly. The in-between phase, that mysterious time when the caterpillar is no longer a caterpillar but not yet a butterfly, can be thought of as a dark night of the soul; we'll experience these proverbial wildfires many times throughout our one life.

If we trust those times of darkness as necessary passageways on our journey toward growth, we can relax and even come to enjoy the descent. Like a tree, we can root into the earth, into the depth of our experience, and receive what it is that we need. We can walk through the fire with more courage and grace, rather than exhausting ourselves, trying to keep everything the same. Like the maturing chrysalis, when we rest into the deep knowing that the dark is here to nurture and evolve us, we begin to grow our wings.

Stoke the Digestive Fire

Like the caterpillar's descent into the dark to become the butterfly, the process of digestion is itself a sort of dissolution, a breakdown to break through. The food we eat is broken down; the outer form dissolves, so that the energy within the food can be assimilated by our physical body and transmuted as needed. In Ayurveda (the sister science of yoga), the digestive fire is called *agni*, and much attention is given to keeping our digestive fires burning strongly.

It is understood in Ayurveda that if your *agni* (digestive fire)

Chapter Eight

isn't burning brightly, toxins will accumulate in the body (known as *ama*), blocking the flow of creative energy in our whole system (Shakti). If our physical apparatus is bogged down with unprocessed foods, emotions, and experiences, we'll miss out on the magic of life. It is up to us to stoke our digestive fire, to draw nourishment from the food we eat, the conversations we have, and the challenges we go through. We are the only ones who can activate our *agni*.

When your *agni* is strong, your body absorbs what it needs and eliminates the rest. What results is that healthy glow that comes from feeding your body, and nourishing your soul. Known as *tejas* in Sanskrit, that alluring radiance comes from being simmered in the fire of life, becoming more refined and flavourful as you journey on. Literally meaning "cooked from within," *tejas* (inner glow) happens when your *agni* (digestive fire) is powerful enough to transform poison into nectar.

Tend to the Heart Fire

When we moved to Bowen Island, we moved into a beautiful house with a real wood-burning fireplace. Up until then, I had only lived in city dwellings with fireplaces that had an on-off switch. For the first time in my thirty years of being alive, I learned what it took to start and keep a fire going. In tending to the fire in my home hearth, I discovered what it meant to tend to my own heart fire. Tending the physical fire of logs became a mirror for the relationship I had with my own soul. The flame, I quickly discovered, is a living, life-giving force that requires deliberate attention if it is to keep burning. In the same way, the light of my soul requires my conscious participation to be ablaze.

We may not think of the relationship we have with our innermost self as a relationship that needs tending. Perhaps it seems odd to treat your soul as you would your most beloved. But like a fire, the soul is a living presence that needs attention. As Marion Woodman said, "The soul may be forgotten, but never dies." The soul is what enlivens the body. Knowing and bringing that part of you into all that you do is part of your *raison d'être* your reason for being. As long as you have a body, it is not too late to begin to cultivate an enlivening relationship with your innermost self. If you do, your life will take on a fresh new perspective and depth of meaning that you never dreamed possible. If you do not, your soul will use any means necessary to get your attention.

The Beauty Way

"Internally, the mind becomes coarse and dull if it remains unvisited by images and thoughts which hold the radiance of beauty. Even, and perhaps especially in the bleakest times, we can still discover and awaken beauty; these are precisely the times when we need it most. Nowhere else can we find the joy that beauty brings." John O'Donohue

In the same way I learned to tend the fire in my new home, I discovered what it meant to cultivate a relationship with my soul. When I began to understand what fed my particular soul (nature, solitude, deep beauty, laughter, Paris), I became much more intentional about bringing more of these elements into my life. Fresh flowers, loving friendships, and walks in the forest all became daily rituals, part of my return to wholeness and health. The road to rebuilding my malleable clay body after the devastation of chemotherapy and radiation was imbued with a newfound sense of artistry and fun. Instead of doubting my body's ability to heal herself, I began listening to what she really needed. The answer often surprised me. It wasn't only the

Chapter Eight

craving for healthy food or rest that she wanted, but the desire to feel joy again; to feel a spark and love for life. I began buying myself fresh flowers, decorating my home elegantly, wearing colours that enlivened me. I would even wear red lipstick around the house, as a spiritual practice of adorning myself with loving care.

Along with nature, the other most nourishing superfood for the soul is beauty. Not simply the superficial image of perfection we've been entranced to believe is beautiful by our culture, but the deep radiance inherent in all things. The exquisite scent of a rose, the unique feeling of a place, the sparkle in your child's eyes, that note in your favourite song, the lines of a life well-lived etched on a human face. Beauty is everywhere, if we have the eyes to see it. And learn to see it we must, for as John O'Donohue said, "The human soul is hungry for beauty, we seek it everywhere.... We feel most alive in the presence of the Beautiful for it meets the needs of the soul."

Beauty feeds the soul the way food sustains the physical body. Beauty can be seen, smelt, felt, heard, and tasted. It's what awakens us to the joy of being alive. If we only struggle through life and ignore the importance that beauty plays in the vitality of our being, then we'll quickly burn out, become dull, dried out, and brittle. Yet nothing about living an ensouled life is dry. Although meeting our soul can initially happen through wildfires, cocoon times, hardship, and pain, the encounter itself is a loving one, full of allure and wonder.

It can be said that beauty keeps everything alive. The gorgeous vibrant pink cherry blossoms that attract the honey bees do so to keep creation happening. The bees a blossom will attract will go on to pollinate other flowers and plants, which will grow the fruits and become a major food source for many species, including humans. We now know that we could not survive without our vanishing bees, which means we cannot survive without beauty. At the heart of our creative nature is the longing to create beauty through all that we do. Beauty is not a decadent indulgence reserved for the elite and privileged few, but a sacred thread that we must follow if we are to enliven our soul, heal ourselves, and our planet.

The Beauty Way is following the stirrings of the heart. It is following the call of beauty, the sacred thread that guides us each on our journey. It is being deliberate about how we gaze out at the world, choosing to see the beauty in all things. It is not a way to deny the suffering and pain that exist, but to enliven the essence, to digest the delicious nourishment of every moment. The Beauty Way will look different for each of us because in essence, it is the Be You way.

Cultivate Radiance

If the radiance we innately seek comes from being *svastha*, established in the essence of who we are, then vibrant health is a manifestation of a loving relationship we have with our innermost self. Like a tree's root system moves down into the earth to nourish and support its outward flourishing, we must continually tap into the inner wellspring of soul to guide us on our journey to flowering ourselves.

The importance of healthy habits is a well-versed topic in yoga and Ayurveda. Both systems of healing recognize that the little things we do every day lead to greater shifts over time. Although the wildfires in our life will often create rapid change in a short period of time, real transformation and true healing come from how we choose to move forward after such cataclysmic events. How shall we rise from the ashes? Do we allow unpredictable circumstances to control our trajectory? Or can we claim our sovereignty in the face of adversity?

Chapter Eight

Does the fire devour you, pull you into a downward spiral of hopelessness and despair, or does it spark within you desire for and newfound clarity of the kind of life you want to live while you're here?

To cultivate is to devote oneself to promoting growth of one form or another. In Ayurveda, *dinacharya* ("daily ritual") is a daily morning routine designed to clear ourselves of toxicity (*ama*) and increase our innate radiance (*tejas*). Built into daily living is the recognition that you are an energetic being, a light source that must be tended to in order to shine. Like washing windows to see the outside more clearly, *dinacharya* cleanses not only the physical body of toxins, but also the energetic (*pranic*) body, and emotional-mental body (*manas*) of undigested experiences. When your energetic, emotional and mental body hygiene is maintained, it's easier to make choices that reflect the radiance of who you really are.

A seasoned gardener knows that if a rose bush is to flourish, it must be pruned over and over again. Otherwise, the rose bush will produce more roses than it can sustain. If we don't cut it back, the bush won't be able to support all the roses, and one by one they will begin to shrivel up. On a daily basis, we are inundated with information, obligations, and shiny invitations that pull our attention outward. In this digital age of constant connection, we must make a deliberate choice to place our attention and spend our time on pursuits and practices that nurture and nourish the soul. We must learn to say NO unapologetically to all the commitments that do not align with our soul's essential work. We must trim away the excess projects, artificial foods, and perceived responsibilities that weigh us down; they are damp logs that stifle our inner light.

Reflecting on why, as a flight attendant, I instructed people to don their own oxygen mask before helping others, I've come to understand that it is absolutely essential. Fire needs air to burn.

Wildfire Within

You need to keep your own life force ignited if you are to be a source of light for anyone else.

As an agent for transformation, the fire element can teach us how to tend to our own life force. Only we can choose how to engage with the energy of fire. Every day, we must deliberately tend to the fire of our own heart. In this busy age, it won't just happen on its own. We can ignore the flicker, but we can never extinguish the flame. Our Divine birthright and sacred responsibility is to tend to this sacred flame we alone carry. Day by day, choice by choice, we can either blow on the embers of our dreams and deepest desires or stifle our spark with busy schedules and outdated ideas of who we think we are. A line from Oriah Mountain Dreamer's *The Invitation* says it best: "I want to know if you can disappoint another to be true to yourself. If you can bear the accusation of betrayal and not betray your own soul."

We must learn to see ourselves as holy fire tenders, butterfly growers, and blossoming rose gardeners, gifted with the sacred task of flowering our own soul.

Weave Thyself

One of my first tantric philosophy teachers, Douglas Brooks said that "freedom is not having whatever you want, whenever you want. True freedom," he said, "is choosing to want what you already have." As someone who has suffered from FOMO (fear of missing out) for a long time, it was a potent reminder for me to know that I am so free that I can choose to want what I already have.

In Sanskrit, the word for freedom is *svatantrya*. Literally translated as "self-looming," true freedom is not about gaining infinite fame and fortune, even though this is the promise of our consumerist culture, including of yoga. Do this, then you

Chapter Eight

will be happy, buy this product, and all your problems will be solved, then one day at some future time, you'll be free. We're led to believe that once we get rid of the cancer, the debt, the sadness in our heart, then we'll taste true freedom.

I do believe yoga to be a deeply healing path that can help revitalize the body and alleviate the suffering we all sometimes feel as a result of being alive. At times, retail therapy soothes my sorrows and makes me feel happy for a little while. Each therapy has its place. The problem occurs when we mistake the "highs" as the goal, when we think our anger or sadness are problems to be overcome, rather than symptoms of being alive and feeling life deeply. When we mistakenly believe that freedom is about being able to do whatever we want, whenever we want (and to hell with anyone who tries to get in our way), we embark on a sort of spiritual bypass, a hedonistic treadmill chasing only the good stuff in life. You may feel temporary relief when everything in life is going well, but if you're chasing a perpetual high in the name of freedom, then eventually, when things change, as they inevitably always do, the fall will be much greater.

Because our innermost nature is one of unbounded joy and freedom, as humans we are always seeking to recreate that freedom outside ourselves. We spend so many resources lining things up on the outside, not realizing that the freedom and joy we all seek comes from an inner attunement; aligning inwardly to who we really are. Freedom is about remembering that every breath is a gift. It is trusting that life is happening for us, not to us, and knowing that we always have the freedom to choose how to weave ourselves in the greater tapestry of life. Freedom for freedom's sake is an unattainable goal. It is not something you can earn, achieve, or save up for. Rather, freedom is a natural by-product of aligning with your true nature. Freedom happens when you consciously align with your soul and allow it to flow forth, weaving it into the fabric of your life.

As Christopher "Hareesh" Wallis, says in his book *Tantra Illuminated*, "Freedom means actually experiencing the divinity in each moment." It is being present with life, in its full spectrum of colour, experience, and emotions, and not wishing it to be any different.

Freedom is not a result of your external circumstances. The elation of liberation comes from embodying your soul.

The freedom I so desperately sought from a life-threatening illness, a difficult marriage, and the responsibilities of parenthood would not be attained by leaving it all behind and running away from my life. Wherever it was I could run to, I would also bring myself with me. After months of struggle, wishing I had someone else's life, it finally dawned on me that freedom is an inside job. It comes from setting roots inward, grounding down into the depths of my vibrant essence and embracing who I am.

To become truly liberated, I had to actively love myself and my life exactly as they were. I had to see my circumstances not as obstacles to my freedom, but as the very means by which I could remember that I am always already free. We always have the power to see life as happening for us, not to us, and we are free to choose how to walk through this miraculous journey.

Cross the Threshold

As Joseph Campbell famously said, "Follow your bliss and doors will open where there were no doors before." The bliss that he speaks of is that feeling of freedom that arises when you follow the call of your own soul, when you walk your own true way.

Because consciousness informs matter, when we remember our free agency in any given moment, we begin to see possibilities opening up around us, doors opening where there were none before. In yoga mythology, Ganesha is the

Chapter Eight

elephant-headed gatekeeper known as the remover of obstacles. Paradoxically, he is also the one who places the obstacles on the path. Traditionally, he is placed at the threshold or doorway, symbolizing the invitation of seeing every obstacle as a doorway to enter ourself more fully. The obstacles are not meant to stop or thwart our growth. They are there to accelerate our expansion, and recalibrate us to the freedom we already possess.

I recently listened to an interview explaining that as humans, we have the notion of freedom backwards. We think we must have all the right things, then we'll be able to do what we really want, and then we'll be happy. Instead, the speaker (whose name I don't remember) suggested that we must flip the equation and; turn the elusive have-do-be formula into be-do-have. We all seek freedom because it's in an aspect of our true nature. We must remember that we already are free (be); we act and live out our life as though we're choosing all of it (do); and our outer life will become a reflection of our abundant inner alignment (have). The flow of Shakti (creative energy) will be unblocked, and in the same way that a healthy root system nourishes a whole tree, creative energy and power will flow into your mind, heart, body, and your entire life. We must develop a deep enough knowing of our soul nature and see our main taproot as rooting down into nature and soul.

The metaphorical butterfly wings we seek to grow, the freedom we long for, does not come from elevating our vibration to some higher, better place or changing the external conditions of our life. Rather, true freedom arises when we learn to embrace the present moment exactly as it is, to choose what we have. When we stop resisting what is, we lean into our life, and can learn to cherish the beauty of every moment. In welcoming the Mystery, we nourish our soul, and in so doing, grow deeper roots. By embracing the dark, we free up our natural creative energy and liberate our light; we grow wings. The descent always precedes the ascent. Freedom happens when we embody who we really are.

Your Life Is Your Craft

To be *svatantrya*, a liberated self-weaver, is to remember that you carry a thread that is yours alone to carry, your soul's unique radiance. Freedom is consciously choosing how to weave yourself into the fabric of life. Every choice we make is a way to exercise our innate freedom, to participate in the unfolding of our life. We may not be able to choose what comes our way, but we can always choose what meaning to make of it.

Your words become your world.

Four years after my cancer treatments ended, I was out celebrating a girlfriend for her birthday. Among her guests that evening was Danielle LaPorte, one of my favourite authors, someone whose work empowered me greatly during some of my darkest days. As we sat around sipping martinis and peppermint tea, the birthday girl expressed how grateful she was that we were each in her life. We shared laughs and tears over that year's triumphs and trials, and at some point in the night, the "c" bomb was dropped. The girls whom I was meeting for the first time that night were floored to learn that I had gone through a "cancer chapter" only a few years earlier. My luscious long hair and revived twinkle in my eye made it hard to imagine that I had been a cancer patient, not long before.

"So you're okay now?" one of the girls hesitantly asked.

"Yes, I'm in remission going on four years now," I replied.

"Cheers to that!" exclaimed the birthday girl raising her glass. We all joined in for an exuberant "to life!" cheers.

After taking a celebratory sip, we lowered our glasses and Danielle turned to me and lovingly asked: "Let me ask you something. Why do you say you're in remission, and not 'I'm cured?'"

Chapter Eight

"Well ..." I paused, wondering the same thing in that moment. "The doctors say you're really only cured if the cancer never comes back, and the oncologists don't like to say you're cured until you've been in remission for at least five year, so...."

"Fuck that," she interrupted slyly, exuding her rebelliously mystical nature, "it's not coming back, honey. You're cured—start saying so!" She raised her glass for another lively "cheers!" We all joined in: "to being cured!"

In yoga, the power of words is known as Matrika Shakti, *matrika* meaning "little mother." The power of speech is recognized as a creative act. Your words become your world. Like little mothers, the vibrations you birth shape the material plane. From that day forward, I decided that the cancer isn't coming back. Instead of hoping for the best, I reclaimed my power to author my experience of life, and declared myself cured. Through yoga and quantum physics, we know that consciousness affects matter. So do thoughts and words. The way we choose to see ourselves and how we speak about ourselves and others shapes our experience and the material world around us. Your life is your craft, may you weave it beautifully.

More Soul Alignment, Less Daily Grind

When we remember that we are already free and that we alone must decide how to channel our individual life force, we become more present to the magic of life and we begin to notice that we are always being guided.

As I continued to consciously cultivate a loving relationship with my soul, gorgeous opportunities started to appear. It seemed the more rooted I became in my own truth, the more possibilities emerged before me. One such serendipitous event was when I was asked to teach a private class to *New York Times* estselling author, Gabrielle Bernstein. I had admired Gabby's

Wildfire Within

work for years and was elated to be meeting her in person. Before driving to Whistler for our private session, I purchased and downloaded her latest book *The Universe Has Your Back*. As I listened to her audio book driving up the beautiful Sea to Sky Highway, I was struck with the relevance of her teachings. It felt as though she had written the book just for me.

In it, she speaks of paying attention to the recurring signs and symbols that appear in your life. They are signposts from spirit and guidance from the Universe, who always has our highest good in mind. "Pay particular attention to numbers in sequence," she read. "When you see ones in sequence, as in one hundred eleven, it is a sign of Divine guidance, letting you know you are on the right path." At that exact moment, I looked down at the clock and it was 11:11 a.m.! I was blown away at the perfection of life, the sacred synchronicity of it all. Later that day, I shared the story with Gabby and she couldn't believe it. We connected over our shared love of soul symbols, and have stayed in touch ever since. Later that year, I was over joyed when I discovered that the address for my amazing publisher Julie Salisbury at the time of signing this book deal was 111 Beach Street. I could never have orchestrated life perfectly enough to make that happen! The Universe does indeed have our back. And so does our soul.

When we begin to consciously align with our soul, we start to see all the beautiful ways that life is guiding us. Our task is not to figure it all out or to rid ourselves of all our problems. I believe that the freedom we seek comes from surrendering to the path our soul is here to experience. What we really need is less hustle and more Grace. Less self-doubt and more souls come to life. Less worry and more trust in the grand tapestry, and in the sacredly unique thread you alone carry.

CHAPTER NINE

Flourish: Bloom Wildly (Full Moon)

Full Moon: Shine, play, dance, rise, be passionate, love, celebrate, forgive

"Once Awakened, Shakti always Rises." Sally Kempton

"Love is what's left when you let go of all the things you love." Swami Jnaneshvara Bharati

"Don't ask what the world needs. Ask what makes you come alive, and go do it. Because what the world needs is people who have come alive." Howard Thurman

The Full Moon Always Returns

As the moon cycles through her counterclockwise rotation around the earth, she returns to the fullness, from which she never really departed. Although the moon appears to wax and wane, it is all a play of light, a movement of energy. Her true nature is always full, whole, complete unto herself, and her radiance comes from the culmination of all her phases. Her monthly journey into darkness reminds us that all life needs rest and incubation. It is from this space that new life and dreams are born. Seeds root into the dark to grow, bud, and bloom fully. Symbolically, the Full Moon embodies the energy of the full bloom. To truly flourish is not about being busy or successful by our culture's standards, but about grounding into the earth and sharing the light born within.

The Dark Feminine

In the wisdom traditions of the Dark Feminine, destruction always precedes new creation. The Dark Feminine is the less-celebrated yet revitalizing face of the mother. She is Lilith, Kali, Mary Magdalene, and Persephone; she is nighttime and mid-winter. The healing power of awakened sexuality, rage, passion, seduction, courage, and strength are her gifts. She rises from the dead and is comfortable with the true alchemical nature of turning base metal into gold. The Dark Feminine exists to destroy everything that we are not, so we can live into our full potential. Exiled and demonized for centuries, she is often feared and misunderstood. But the Dark Feminine is a deeply loving force who will not let us play small in a world that needs our radiance. She reminds us that times of chaos and dissolution give way to new life and new possibilities. Death is always followed by rebirth and, as much as we'd love to, we can't skip over the dying part.

On a cellular level, cancer is an inability to die. It manifests when the cell's expiration date ceases to exist. When the cell goes on growing, consuming, and devouring everything in its path, it blocks the natural flow of life. It creates excess, unsustainable growth. Cancer happens when the cell forgets how to let go and let flow.

In a way, we humans have become like cancerous cells that have forgotten our rightful place in nature and with each other.

Chapter Nine

We have disremembered how to be in right relationship with all that is. Under the delusion of "more is better," inwardly reciting "me, me, me" as our mantra, we have caused much damage to ourselves, and to our planet. By believing that unbounded material growth is the goal and key to happiness, we have created dis-ease in ourselves and in our world.

On my own journey to healing, I had to let go and let die old ways of being and moving through life. Through the crucible of motherhood and cancer, my spiritual journey transformed into one of descent and embrace, rather than one of ascension and perfection. By viewing my predicament as an initiation, I remembered my capacity to adapt and evolve in the face of devastation. Cancer became a liberating catalyst. It was my soul's cry, a call to stop living in a way that denied her existence. Cancer was not a malignant intruder sent forth to ruin my life; it was a Divine messenger, an indicator of my body's deep intelligence.

Before cancer, I thought that being healthy came from eating the right food, thinking the right thoughts, and being kind to others. I truly believed that if I did all the right things, I would reach a place of perfection and be vibrationally shielded from hardships, and become immune to life's pain. But in the purifying heat of the cancer fire, I realized that what I needed to change in my life was not my lifestyle; what I ate and what kind of work I was doing. My path to healing was about transmuting my relationship to myself and to all of life. Cancer for me was a radical recalibration from within and, as are all moments of chaos in life, opportunities for deeper alignment with oneself.

In seeking to return to health, I embarked on a journey back to wholeness. What I discovered was all the ways I had been living a partial existence. By living a goal- oriented life, excessively focused on doing and achieving rather than being and feeling, I had exiled the Divine feminine within me. In trying to attain everlasting happiness, spiritual mastery, and perfection, I had malnourished my soul, mistreated my body, and condemned the playfully wild and wise woman within me.

Subconsciously I had fallen for the delusion that I needed to earn joy and freedom, that happiness lay elsewhere, any place other than this very breath. I began to realize that in seeking to control the circumstances of my life, the love I had for myself and for others became very conditional. By trying to be spiritual, I suppressed everything within me which was "not spiritual." Anger, disappointment, sadness were forced to go underground, rather than simply flowing through or providing useful feedback. Since it was too painful to feel the discomfort of suppressed emotions, I shut down internally, silencing my voice, ignoring my intuition, and cutting myself off from an inner wellspring of wisdom, joy, and deep beauty.

By trying to keep my vibration high by avoiding any negativity, I pacified conflict and numbed myself, attempting to fit into everyone else's version of spirituality. Pleasing others and avoiding anything unpleasant became my new religion in the name of kindness and service and love. In trying to make others happy and keep myself buoyed up all the time, I muted my authentic connection to source and cut myself off from my own power. I discounted the rejuvenating darkness of sleep, sadness, and winter. I believed my mind to be more intelligent than my body and ignored the internal guidance of my soul.

When chemo treatments ended and I began learning about the rhythms of nature, the soulful heroine's journey, and the cycles of the moon, I started to feel the incredible power and eternal presence of the sacred feminine. I realized that my early quest to grow spiritually came from a desire to transcend death, from a lack of self-worth, and a disregard for nature. On a deep level, I believed that I needed to change and perfect myself before I could truly be free and deeply lovable. It came

Chapter Nine

from a place of lack, a feeling of not being enough just as I was. My desire to grow resembled the quest for some Holy Grail, a search for completion that would never come. Ironically and paradoxically, the Holy Grail symbolizes the Divine feminine, so I found her in the end, within myself. And she was not what I expected. The grail as the chalice also represents the creative flow of the Divine feminine, and so will never cease to create. There is no final destination at which to arrive, but only the gift of the journey itself.

In coming to understand all the ways I had ignored the Divine feminine within myself, I knew that what I needed for my body to return to its natural state of health was a return to wholeness, a reclamation of the Divine feminine. To be healthy, I had to embrace and embody parts of myself that I had ignored. To truly blossom from a place of wholeness, I had to drink from the overflowing well that was my very own experience.

Remember to Remember

After the wildfire of cancer, new motherhood, and the breakdown of my marriage, the landscape of my life was unrecognizable. No longer the globe-trotting, innocent maiden of my youth, I found myself in a completely new realm of reality. Although the outer terrain of my daily life had been transfigured by the flames, within me was ignited that which was true and lasting. The essence of me, my soul, had been consecrated by fire, fortified, purified, and made stronger and more vibrant by the experience. Living a soul-driven life was no longer a wishful intention or theoretical concept. It was the only way to survive and truly thrive. Through rediscovering all the ways I had exiled the sacred feminine within and around me, cancer was teaching me that the only way out was through a radical embrace of myself and my life, exactly as I was, without the need to fix or change a thing. To heal, I needed to let go of control, open myself to spirit, and love without condition.

As I began to release my grip on things needing to be a certain way before I could let my innate joy flow, I started to re-member who I am. Like blowing softly on the embers of my true self, my inner knowing grew in brightness and clarity. I was not a cancer patient, a yoga teacher, a mother, or any of the other roles that I occupied for a time. These were but labels I wore like a wardrobe. Who I was, who I was becoming, who I am is a creative embodied soul, here to experience and express the fullness of life. Through the many roles that I will play, I am here to weave meaning and create beauty from my experiences, and to expand my capacity to love.

We are each meant to shine in the particular way we were uniquely crafted to emanate light. As the late Richard Wagamese once wrote, "Remember to remember." To heal, I needed to put myself back together; to literally re-member myself, and embody the luminosity from which I came.

Today, five years since being diagnosed with cancer, I can look back and truly see how my life has been enriched by the wildfire that destroyed and saved me, simultaneously. As I learned to call back the fragmented parts of myself and embody the truth of who I am, my life has continued to flourish in unexpected ways. Greg and I have learned to embrace the messiness of our humanity, and we support each other in blossoming our souls. Not only did I emerge from the ashes revitalized and strengthened, but our relationship did too. As we give each other the gift of our attention, presence, and care, as we learn to cherish and nourish each other, our relationship continues to flourish. We've built a beautiful life here on Bowen Island, surrounded by majestic cedars and the Pacific Ocean; we have become deeply rooted in nature and community. Benjamin runs wild through the forests and loves to bathe in the sea. We

Chapter Nine

still have our issues and life will always have its challenges, but I've come to learn that that is part of the fun of being here. The fullness of the experience is what makes it such a wildly fulfilling ride.

Perfectly Imperfect

To navigate daily life and understand our place in it, we like to label things as "good" and "bad." We spend a lot of energy avoiding the bad in order to make room for more good. We think of some emotions as negative and others as positive, creating a false hierarchy and a sense of separation between movements of energy. We deem getting married and making money as "good," and see falling ill or breaking up as "bad." Rather than putting everything into neat piles of "this is good" and "that is bad," tantra recognizes instead that within every experience, there is a little bit of both: some good and some bad.

The tantric view invites us to see things as either "beneficial" to our growth or not. Rather than classifying things as "good" or "bad," tantra is more concerned about how we utilize the energy inherent in every experience, how we churn poison to nectar and draw forth nutrients for our soul's expansion. Every contraction leads to a greater expansion, and anything that happens can be transformed into life-giving compost. In every moment, we can choose to create healing by integrating what we've learned, re-wholing ourselves. Or, we can use any experience to justify more separation, creating a larger tear in the tapestry. *Tantrikas* (those who view life through the tantric lens) believe that we are not inherently good or bad but, rather, we carry the potential to create it all. Within each of us is the whole spectrum. As above, so below; the entire Universe is inside.

The goal of tantra then is not to perfect or purify yourself to some heightened state. The aim of tantra rather is to remind you that you are already innately whole—like the moon, you are already and always full, but only appear otherwise as you cycle through the many facets and phases of wholeness. Through it all, you are the master weaver, free to spin the stories and piece together the twists and turns into the great tapestry that becomes your life. Will you pay attention, hold to, and pull through the threads that truly matter, weaving more beauty in the world? Or will you randomly react as you go, aimlessly creating knots around your heart, adding to the confusion and chaos?

To be healthy means to be whole. It means to cherish and nourish all levels of your being. It is knowing that the earth, your body, heart, and soul are all necessary parts of the whole. Winter, rest, inward reflection, and times of apparent stillness are required pieces of the full, healthy life pie. You cannot simply live as though you have a mind or a body, and deny nourishment to your soul. You can't live a life of spirit and ignore the divinity of your body. You cannot walk upon the earth as though you are above nature, but must come to know yourself as a conscious expression of the earth herself and, at the same time, as an embodiment of spirit. You are the meeting point, the dwelling place where spirit and matter converge, the bridge between the worlds, the midwife for creativity and change. To truly be healthy, you must learn to inhabit and integrate all parts of your Self.

Our true nature is *purnatva*, perfectly imperfect, wholeness from which can arise infinite potential. To be healthy is to be life-enhancing and generative. It is to embrace the whole of yourself, and consciously create that which you desire to see in the world.

Chapter Nine

Created to Create

"Your Suppressed Creativity is not benign." Brené Brown

Whether you identify yourself as a "creative" person or not, you are born a creatrix, here to move, respond, weave, and participate in the unfolding of your life. As an embodiment of spirit, creativity is part of your innate wiring. If you suppress the natural nudge to create, it will metastasize as resentment or anger. Unexpressed desires and unlived dreams will lodge themselves in the crevices of your heart and body, creating uncomfortable aches, disguising themselves as anxiety, stress, or depression. Do not let these pathologies of soul take root inside you. See, feel, and respect these inner longings. Free yourself from the discomfort of misplaced power by reclaiming your creative spirit.

By creativity, I am not solely refereeing to your artistic abilities or peripheral playtime pursuits. Your creativity is the way you respond to life. It is your natural aptitude to dream and envision a new way of being. It is the freedom to choose how to show up, how to view life, and how to make meaning out of it all. Creativity is remembering that we are all born storytellers; we are each crafting our own personal mythology and authoring our own experience. It is the impulse to grow, to thrive, and to flourish. We have survived and evolved as a species, because we are created to create.

If creativity is central to who we are, then it is also closely tied to our health and vitality. When we make space in our day to be creative for its own sake, we experience lowered cortisol (stress) levels and higher levels of serotonin. We get high on being creative. It is not frivolous. On the contrary, being creative is at the heart of being vibrantly alive. Creating and witnessing beauty, in all its forms, is deep medicine. In our soul-parched society that values breadth over depth, we need to reclaim our innate creativity if we are to quench the thirst that guides us and embody the wellbeing that is our birthright.

Choosing to channel your creativity is giving yourself permission to be who you really are. It's reclaiming your sovereign power as a participant in your own and in the Universe's creation story.

You can be creative in your nine-to-five job, your entrepreneurial project, or at home with your children. The way you prepare and plate a meal, the way you make the bed and rise to greet the day, how you dress yourself and greet your partner, how you write the email and walk the dog are all creative acts. We often get so focused on the desired results of what we're doing that we forget to be in the delight of the dance. This is where true creativity lies, in the secret interior space of your experience.

Although we think of creativity as a form of self-expression, I see it more as an act of worship. It is the relationship you keep with your life force as she moves through your veins and invites you to interact with flare to the various demands of your day.

It is the way you infuse presence into every breath.

There has never been another you on the planet. This day has never before existed. The constellations have never coalesced the same way they do in this moment. Be the conscious maker that you are, living on the frontier of what has never been before. Be willing to see things another way. Respond instead of react, fashion your way forward. Participate in your own becoming. Show up, create, and emanate, the way that only you can.

Your Desires Become Your Destiny

Since we are all born creators, I believe that the unique desires we each carry are not random or whimsical. They

Chapter Nine

are placed within each of us precisely because we are the ones to make them manifest. Desires carry within them the blueprint of our destiny, the seeds for that which we are born to become and here to create.

Over the years, I've had an on-again-off-again type of love affair with my desires. Confused about their purpose and meaning, I often struggled to know what to do with them. Is what I truly desire a distraction from spiritual progress, something to be suppressed and eradicated? Perhaps as some religions suggest, desire is an evil force keeping me running on the hedonistic treadmill, never feeling quite satisfied enough, always reaching for more. Does it even matter what I desire? I've wondered.

At times I knew what I wanted so clearly that it was painful to ignore. Other times, the nebulousness of not knowing what I wanted led to wasting much energy and resenting others. But more painful than knowing and not listening—or just being unsure of what I really wanted—was desiring nothing at all. Total numbness. By this, I am not referring to contentment, where one is so satisfied she longs for nothing (contentment is appreciating every part of the journey and the wellspring from which desire bubbles up). But rather, a total disconnect from the energy of desire, a complete withdrawal from life.

During chemotherapy, before my conscious relationship with the Dark Feminine, I became fearful of life. Feeling let down with a cancer diagnosis, I felt betrayed, and became afraid to trust myself and the wisdom of my body. I was afraid of letting myself be too hopeful or dream too big, fearing that I might not live long enough to see it manifest. It would be less painful, I thought, to just go on living by numbing myself to the desires I carried within me.

That state of being disconnected from the energy of desire was more than just depression; it felt like hell.

With time and a willingness to heal, I allowed myself to feel

Wildfire Within

again the pain of facing my own death and the joy of looking into my son's eyes. When I made the choice to stay awake to the beauty of life, the life spark of desire ignited inside me. I realized that if I was going to make it out alive, I had to want it. And with that, desire became my life force.

The will to live seems like a basic, built-in mechanism to ensure the survival of our species. But as I moved along the spectrum from being terrified of life to really wanting to *live* fully, I recognized that my desires came from a place deeper than my will, my intellect, or my aesthetic preferences. Desire was the loving, intelligent, creative, and generative force pulling me forward, energizing me from within. I started to see my desires as callings from my soul, impulses sent forth as signals, honing mechanisms helping me distil how to best utilize and enjoy my time on the planet. Awakening to my desires brought me back to life.

"Follow desire back to its source," my teacher Hareesh would say. What he and all the ancient tantric traditions are pointing to is the inherent, liberating, and self-actualizing power of creative energy.

Rather than focusing on the external object or goal as the "thing" that you desire, they explain, try to identify what you think having that thing, that relationship with that person, or that experience will bring you. Most likely, you'll find that beneath the outer layer of what you want is a deep longing to feel a certain way, to connect with a part of yourself that you forgot was there all along. It's about bringing forth something within you that is ready to wake up.

The word "desire" is from the Latin *desiderare* meaning, "to gaze at the stars." It also shares its roots with the Latin word "to decide" meaning to cut off. Your desires are of the stars, they point to your destiny. When you pay attention and choose to follow where desire wants to take you, you close other doors, and cut yourself off from the possibility of living anything but a life aligned with the stars.

Call it your soul, your essence, the Divine spark within you;

Chapter Nine

it doesn't really matter what you name the unnameable. What matters is that there is an intelligent, loving, and creative force within you here to be seen, felt, and activated. Your desires matter. The world needs you to make your desires manifest. That is why you are here.

Wildfire

"Our deepest fear is not that we are inadequate. Our deepest fear is that we are powerful beyond measure. It is our light, not our darkness that most frightens us. We ask ourselves, 'Who am I to be brilliant, gorgeous, talented, fabulous?' Actually, who are you not to be? You are a child of God. Your playing small does not serve the world. There is nothing enlightened about shrinking so that other people won't feel insecure around you. We are all meant to shine, as children do. We were born to make manifest the glory of God that is within us. It's not just in some of us; it's in everyone. And as we let our own light shine, we unconsciously give other people permission to do the same. As we are liberated from our own fear, our presence automatically liberates others." Marianne Williamson

The wildfire within you is the most natural part of you. It is the light you were born to shine through every moment of your life. The more we embrace and embody who we really are, the more we free those around us to do the same.

In yoga, the heat created by our practice is called *tapas*. Just as rubbing two sticks together creates the necessary tension to ignite a flame, intense experiences in life catalyze our own soul spark. We all experience stress, but it's how we respond to stress that determines whether we burn out or become brighter because of it. *Tapas*—the fire of our will—creates *tejas*, the inner glow that comes from being cooked from within, which emanates from knowing and following your innate resilience to move through life's challenge with courage and tenacity. *Tapas* create *tejas*; fire creates light.

The wildfire within you is a radiant inner force here to expand you. Your soul wants to be expressed and, ultimately, embodied. It is your very nature, luminous and free. If denied, repressed, and suppressed, this most essential part of you will devour you from the inside, leaving you feeling sick, resentful, tired, and uninspired.

If allowed to shine, it will be a powerful and liberating source of light, clearing your path of all the parts of you and your life that you no longer need. Whatever is not really you will be incinerated, leaving more space for your soul flame to shine more brightly. Increasing your inner radiance inspires and frees others to do the same. Like a wildfire, living a soul-centred life catches on. Thoughts, beliefs, and ways of being become stronger when shared.

Redwoods

The year I got married, so did many of our friends, and all three of Greg's siblings. At each of her four children's weddings that year, my mother-in-law read a lovingly crafted speech. Although each of the speeches was as different as her children, there was a common story she shared in all of them. She told us the story of the sequoia tree.

Also known as the redwoods, this family of giant, ancient trees is renowned for its longevity and strength (some individual sequoias live up to 1,500 years). Towering up to three hundred feet aboveground, these grand conifers only grow in groves, intertwining their roots belowground to share resources. They don't need much because they don't compete for sustenance; they feed each other. It is believed that their interdependence

Chapter Nine

is the reason for their remarkable resilience. My mother-in-law shared this story to illustrate the incredible power of family, community, and support systems. There are many details that have become a blur since my wedding day, but the magical majesty of the sequoias is something I will never forget.

Since then, their symbolism has become even more relevant in my quest to heal the sacred feminine within me. Due to their red bark, they are often referred to as the redwoods, having the same vibrationally rich colour as moon blood, symbolic of Mary Magdalene and the Divine femme. I've since come to understand that their strength comes from their innately feminine qualities to support and nourish, rather than compete and divide. The trees' strength comes from growing together. Soul growth is not an individual occurrence. When one tree is nourished, all other root systems are fed—everyone benefits. We rise together. To thrive and flourish are the most generous things you can do with your one wild and precious life.

Wild Flowers

Comparing the soul's journey to a wildfire is not to deny the fact that transformation and loss are painful parts of existence. Evolution is not an easy process. Neither is childbirth. But we know that the outcome is worth the work.

Since moving to Bowen Island, I have begun teaching yoga at a drug and alcohol treatment centre. Working there has forced me to look at my own addictive tendencies, at all the ways I have numbed myself from feeling whatever it is I really needed to feel. "Hi, my name is Chantal. I'm a recovering perpetual people pleaser, self-help addict, narcissistic perfectionist struggling with pathological positivity."

It is well-understood that most people suffering from addiction have survived multiple forms of trauma throughout their life.

Trauma happens anytime our system is overloaded, overwhelmed, and unable to respond appropriately. Post-traumatic stress disorder (PTSD) has become a modern-day epidemic. Stress is a normal part of everyday life. New research in the field of epigenetics is finding that it's not so much the amount or kind of stress we experience in our life that determines the difference between surviving and truly thriving, but how we respond to the stressful stimulus.

Less well-known is a response to stressful events known as post-traumatic growth (PTG). PTG refers to positive psychological change experienced as a result of adversity and other challenges in order to rise to a higher level of functioning.

To grow post-traumatically, to really thrive after hardship is not merely to bounce back to the shape you once were. It is not only about being resilient and returning to an old way of being. To flourish is to open oneself to the fertile darkness of challenging times, and root into the remembrance that all is happening for you. Every contraction is a precursor to a greater expansion. Fireweed, which flourishes after a wildfire, is known as a pioneer species; it blazes a trail where others dare not yet grow. Like the dandelion emerging and breaking through dense concrete, we can bloom in unexpected places.

Be Your Own Midwife

To know the love of the Dark Goddess is to trust in the power of rebirth. It is understanding that life and time are not linear, but a great spiral dance, a continuum of life, death, and rebirth. To embody the Divine feminine is to realize (to make real) that every death is followed by a rebirth. As women, we are innately created to create life, to receive and to let go. We know deep in our bones that times of crisis are also times of wild creativity, portals of infinite potential from which anything can arise.

Chapter Nine

To awaken and heal the sacred feminine is to reclaim our power to rebirth ourselves and, in so doing, our culture. Rooted in the visions of our hearts' desires, we must become the midwives for change we want to see in the world. To restore the lunar wisdom we so desperately need on our planet at this time, we must remember to keep our hearts wildly attuned to the deeper callings of our souls and bring our whole selves to life.

Savasana

At the end of every yoga class, we practise Savasana or corpse pose. This pose is said to be the most important of all poses. It is designed to offer rest after exertion, and to make space and time for the assimilation and integration of all the benefits of the yoga practice.

Symbolically, Savasana represents not only the end of class, but the end of a life; the completion of a cycle, death. We practise Savasana not only to rest and rejuvenate ourselves after an arduous class, but to practise our own death, consciously. No matter how hard we have practised or how much love we have shared, we will all go through this great transition come the end of our life. In yoga, we practise our death because we recognize it is a natural and inevitable part of daily living. Whether big or small, we will be asked to let go many times throughout the day and throughout our lifetime. Contemplating death is not morbid. On the contrary, it liberates us to live more fully.

In yoga, life force is referred to as *prana*. It's the vital energy that flows through your body, activates your heartbeat, and ignites the twinkle in your eye. Much attention is given to increasing the flow of *prana*, for without it, we'd be but a lifeless bag of bones. But with so much focus on magnifying our life force, we often forget that the most life-enhancing thing we can do is to befriend our own death, to remember the sacred fragility of our

Wildfire Within

time here. The Greek philosophers personified and named this force of nature that devours time and matter Thanatos. Thanatos ("death force") is what makes life force so precious. Without death, life wouldn't be as rich and beautiful and worth savouring.

We must be able to let go of all that we think we are to die unto our old selves, if we are to embody the fullness of who we are. As paradoxical as it may seem, sometimes the "moreness" we seek comes from letting go, letting go of the need to master and control life and letting go of needing things to go a certain way. The more we embrace death force as a constant companion, the more skillful we can become with our sacred life force. We don't take a single breath for granted, remembering that it is all a gift. Without death force, life force would be impotent.

Learn to embrace and dance with the Great Mystery and trust the timing of your life. Just as the seasons happen in their own perfect timing without our interference, so too does our life's unfolding have a natural rhythm. We need not force ourselves to bloom but, rather, we must stop pushing against and resisting the power that wants to expand us.

To let go is not to sit back and become a passive observer in life. To let go is to unravel the knots you have tied around your heart that have kept you from experiencing the joy that is your birthright. To let go is to open up, to feel the breath within the breath. It is to become an active listener, to feel more deeply, to let your presence infuse every moment. To let go is to trust the way Spirit wants to guide you. It is to root into the dark mystery of life in order to flower into who you're here to become. To let go is to choose to release the resistance and be who you're here to be.

Embrace who you are. Liberate your light. Let the Wildfire Within you burn brightly.

Author Biography

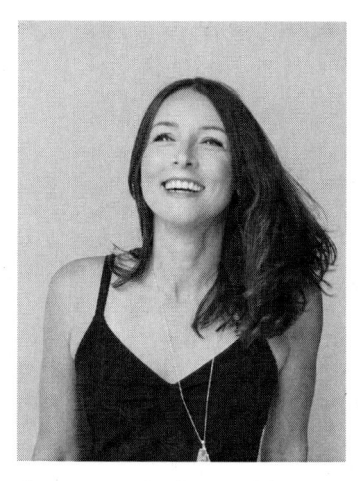

As a mama, entrepreneur, and yogini, Chantal is passionate about living a soul-centred life and is dedicated to awakening the healing power inherent in every human heart. She is a Registered Holistic Nutritionist, a faculty member at The Vancouver School of Yoga, and founder and director of Bowen Island Yoga, located off the West Coast of British Columbia where she resides. Chantal also manages the yoga and nutrition program at The Orchard Recovery Center, teaches workshops throughout Canada and Europe, runs retreats around the world, and is a regular contributor to numerous blogs, including *The Urban Howl*.

When not teaching or writing, she can be found gardening with her husband and son, reading by the fire, or travelling the world in search of good waves, healing foods, and nourishing conversation.

Contact The Author

www.chantalrussell.com
IG: @chantalrussell
Facebook: www.facebook.com/chantal.russell.12
me@chantalrussell.com

Appendix 1

the MOON CYCLE

FULL MOON
Shine, play, dance, rise,
be passionate, love,
celebrate, forgive

DISSEMINATING MOON
Gather, relax,
accept, understand,
regroup, wander

GIBBOUS MOON
Clarify, persevere,
ask, design, tweak,
hone, adjust, expand

LAST QUARTER MOON
Listen within,
turn inward,
reevaluate,
reorient toward
letting go

FIRST QUARTER MOON
Activate,
build, risk,
be confident,
plunge in,
promise, commit

BALSAMIC MOON
Let go, trust fate,
meditate, heal,
soothe, rest, breathe

CRESCENT MOON
Step out, mobilize,
hope, have faith,
reach, begin

NEW MOON
Plant, intuit, open,
tell the truth, dream,
surrender, release

Appendix 2

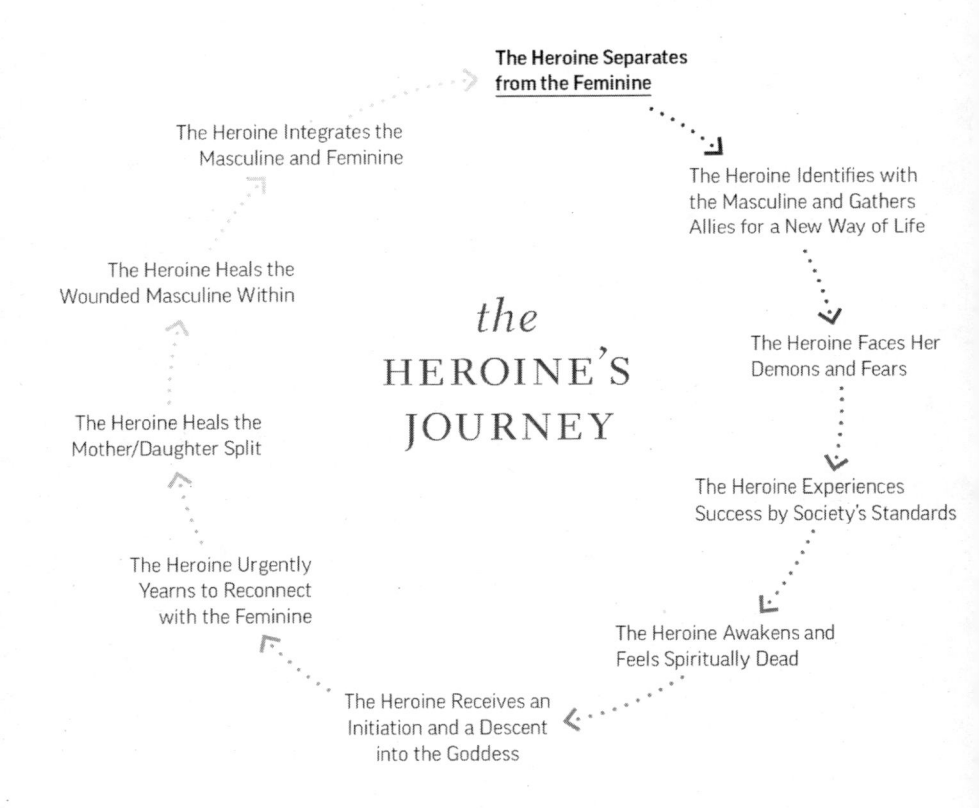

the HEROINE'S JOURNEY

- The Heroine Separates from the Feminine
- The Heroine Identifies with the Masculine and Gathers Allies for a New Way of Life
- The Heroine Faces Her Demons and Fears
- The Heroine Experiences Success by Society's Standards
- The Heroine Awakens and Feels Spiritually Dead
- The Heroine Receives an Initiation and a Descent into the Goddess
- The Heroine Urgently Yearns to Reconnect with the Feminine
- The Heroine Heals the Mother/Daughter Split
- The Heroine Heals the Wounded Masculine Within
- The Heroine Integrates the Masculine and Feminine

Source: Murdock, M. (1990). *The Heroine's Journey: Woman's Quest for Wholeness*. Boston: Shambhala Pub.

Appendix 3

THE KOSHAS
The Five Sheaths

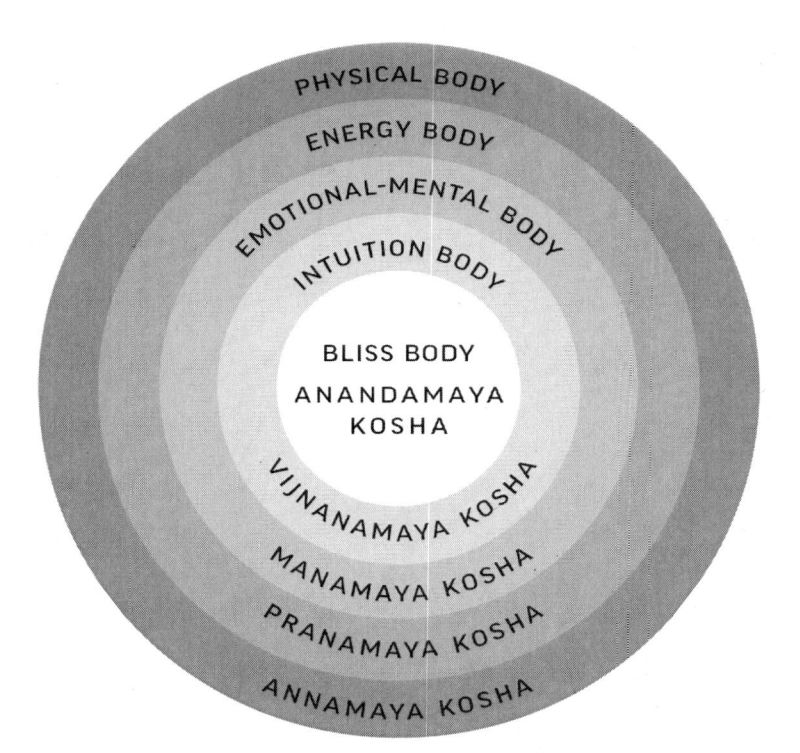

- PHYSICAL BODY
- ENERGY BODY
- EMOTIONAL-MENTAL BODY
- INTUITION BODY
- BLISS BODY
  ANANDAMAYA KOSHA
- VIJNANAMAYA KOSHA
- MANAMAYA KOSHA
- PRANAMAYA KOSHA
- ANNAMAYA KOSHA